RENEWALS 458-4574

DATE DUE

GAYLORD			PRINTED IN U.S.A.

A GUIDE TO METHODS IN THE BIOMEDICAL SCIENCES

A GUIDE TO METHODS IN THE BIOMEDICAL SCIENCES

RONALD B. CORLEY, Ph.D.
Boston University School of Medicine
Boston, MA, USA

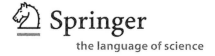
Springer
the language of science

Ronald B. Corley
Boston University School of Medicine
Department of Microbiology
715 Albany Street, L504
Boston, MA 02118
USA
rbcorley@bu.edu

Library of Congress Cataloging-in-Publication Data

Corley, Ronald B.
    A Guide to Methods in the Biomedical Sciences / Ronald B. Corley.
        p.   cm.
    Includes index.
    ISBN 0-387-22844-6   e-ISBN 0-387-22845-4   Printed on acid-free paper.
    1. Medical sciences—Research—Methodology.   I. Title

R855.3.C67 2004
610′.72—dc22   2004056521

Printed in the United States of America.

9 8 7 6 5 4 3 2 1   SPIN 11052234

springeronline.com

*Thanks to TLOML GOMD
and to all of our children, to whom I dedicate this.*

Acknowledgements

There are many people to thank for their help in making this book possible. A true debt of gratitude goes to the many students and technicians who have worked in my laboratory, and made bringing new methods to the lab so much fun. I have learned more from you than you did from me. You would never have known that some of your work would end up in a book like this! Thanks also to Alex for help with research, Kylle for all the proofreading, Kateri for help with the figures, and Kathy for bailing me out as needed.

Contents

Introduction

Students often remark to me how difficult it is to begin reading the primary, journal based literature or follow lectures in a biomedical discipline without some understanding of the methods being used. I can certainly understand their dilemma. While learning "the facts" in science does not necessarily require a working knowledge of HOW we arrive at a conclusion (though it certainly helps!), it is a very different process to begin to understand how we know what we know, and what the limitations of that knowledge might be. This requires first a basic understanding of the methods used to achieve that knowledge, which is followed later by a more detailed and sophisticated understanding of the nuances of the techniques used. In addition, because the tools of science are rapidly evolving, even sophisticated students (and faculty for that matter) can be challenged when beginning to read in a new discipline, where a whole new language emerges.

And, if it is difficult for students, it must be equally frustrating for the lay public to figure out how things are done. To be sure, it is not just students who should be interested in scientific methodology. The use of biomedical techniques is exploding in everyday life: from pregnancy and paternity testing to genetic testing for fetal development, tracing ancestry, and forensics, to new antibody based diagnostic procedures, it is hard to live in today's society and not be touched directly or indirectly by many of the same methods that are used in a biomedical laboratory.

So, how does a student new to science (or an interested lay person) begin to learn the language of techniques? Usually, s/he asks a faculty member, or a colleague, in hopes they might help. Or, the student might scan the web in hopes of obtaining quick (and accurate) information. Or, if they have access to a laboratory, they might consult a classic techniques manual such as the "Red Book" (some excellent methods manuals are listed at the end of the book). However, methods manuals generally provide far more information than necessary at the beginning. Their sheer size can make simply leafing through one of these manuals a daunting task. My students have often said that they would like to have available a simple "pocket primer" describing some of the essential techniques, giving just enough information to get started, but not so much information to bury them in the details.

The purpose of this book is to attempt to meet that need, filling the void between no information and too much detail. It is intended to provide a basic description of common methodology, identify the type of information that can be obtained from a particular technique and, when appropriate, provide alternative approaches. I have always found the history of science interesting, so where possible I have included some historical background to the development of particular techniques. Significant scientific advances rarely occur without the development of new and exciting techniques that can be applied to solving problems. A number of technical advances were of sufficient value to earn for their discoverers a Nobel Prize and many major advances were accompanied by the development of new techniques. I have included some of these breakthroughs in this book as well, and provided where I thought appropriate the original references for some of these major discoveries.

But what techniques should be included? There are thousands of methods that have been developed in the various biomedical disciplines, and if the book was to remain compact the methods included would have to be limited in some way. In deciding on what these might be, I have had numerous discussions with faculty colleagues and students who have provided me excellent suggestions. In the end, I felt that to be the most useful that I would limit the methods not only to those that are frequently used, but to those used in several different disciplines as well. I have also divided the book into 6 basic sections to highlight the selected methods in protein chemistry, nucleic acids, recombinant DNA, antibody-based techniques, microscopy and imaging, and the use of animals in biomedical sciences. I also added a subsection on forensics, and tossed in a few other techniques that I thought would be of interest. In the end, I decided on which techniques "made the cut" (no, they were not selected solely on the basis of whether I've used them in my lab), and the organization of the book reflects what is probably my own idiosyncratic way of thinking. I think most of the basic methods are covered, but if you think a method that should have been included is not, let me know!

Chapter 1

DETECTION AND ANALYSIS OF PROTEINS

A.   Introduction

Proteins are the body's building blocks. They are the second most abundant part of our bodies, comprising about 20% of our weight (the most abundant constituent, water, accounts for 70%). Proteins make up muscles, most of our enzymes are proteins, and the antibodies that protect us from pathogens are glycoproteins, or proteins that also contain carbohydrate sidechains. Proteins are biopolymers that consist of various mixtures of the 20 amino acids. The word "protein" is derived from a Greek root meaning "of first importance". Proteins were discovered in 1838 by Jöns Jacob Berzelius (1779–1848), a Swedish chemist. Berzelius also developed a system of chemical notation that is essentially the same basic system used today. Berzelius is one of three chemists who are considered the fathers of modern chemistry. The other two chemists are Antoine Levoisier (1743–1794) and John Dalton (1766–1844). Levoisier was the first to articulate and experimentally demonstrate the idea of the conservation of matter. He used quantitative methods to measure products of chemical reactions, allowing the composition of compounds to be determined with considerable accuracy. Levoisier also had the distinction of losing his head (literally!) during the French Revolution.

John Dalton made numerous contributions to the field of chemistry. He formulated the atomic theory, which proposed that elements were composed of atoms in fixed amounts and, therefore, each element had a fixed mass. His name is inextricably linked to measurements of weights of proteins. The basic unit is a "Dalton", or Da, which is defined as one-twelfth the mass of the most abundant isotope of carbon, ^{12}C, which is equal to $1.66053873 \times 10^{-24}$ grams. The association of Dalton's name with precise measurements of atomic mass seems ironic to me, in that Dalton was said to be a brilliant mind but not a particularly good

Table 1. Selected Nobel Laureates (Protein Chemistry)

Hermann Emil Fischer	structure of biomolecules; proof that protein molecules are chains of amino acids	1902*
Sir William Henry Bragg William Lawrence Bragg	use of x-ray diffraction for structural analysis	1915[†]
Jean Baptiste Perrin	sedimentation equilibrium	1926[†]
Theodor Svedberg	development and use of ultracentrifuge to determine molecular weight	1926*
George de Hevesy	use of isotopes as tracers	1943*
James Batcheller Sumner John Howard Northrop Wendell Meredith Stanley	chrystallography of proteins; protein purification and structure	1946*
Arne W.K. Tiselius	development of electrophoresis and adsorption to analyze proteins in complex mixtures	1948*
Archer John Porter Martin Richard L.M. Synge	development of partition (paper) chromatography	1952*
Linus Carl Pauling	discovery of chemical bonds	1954*
Frederick Sanger	structure and amino acid sequence of insulin	1958*
Max F. Perutz Sir John C. Kendrew	use of x-ray diffraction to solve structure of globular proteins	1962*
Herbert A. Hauptman Jerome Karle	development of methods to directly use x-ray diffraction information to solve structure	1985*
Richard R. Ernst	development of NMR	1991*
John B. Fenn Koichi Tanaka Kurt Wüthrich	structural analysis of macromolecules (mass spectrophoscopy; NMR)	2002*

*Nobel Prize in Chemistry
[†]Nobel Prize in Physics

experimentalist, even to the point of using inaccurate instrumentation for his measurements. But Dalton's curious mind also led him to be the first to identify color blindness, a condition that both he and his brother suffered from. In an attempt to permit the discovery of the molecular basis for his color blindness, he donated his eyes (not his head!) for study upon his death.

The discovery that proteins are composed of strings of amino acids was made by Hermann Fischer, who won the Nobel Prize in Chemistry in 1902 for his accomplishment (Table 1). The amino acids are joined together by peptide bonds, and consequently proteins are often referred to as polypeptides. Peptide bonds form between the carbon atom of the carboxyl group and nitrogen atom of the amino group of adjacent amino acids. The sequence of amino acids make up a protein identifies its primary structure. The primary amino acid structure dictates local folding patterns within individual protein domains that are common to a number of different proteins. These folding patterns form the secondary structure of a protein. Linus Pauling, who won the Nobel Prize in Chemistry in 1954 for describing chemicala bonds, used both experimental approaches as well as models of small polypeptide chains to determine the orientation of the peptide bond. He found that because of the rigidity of the peptide bonds, amino acids would naturally assume common secondary structures stabilized by hydrogen bonds. The most common secondary structures are "beta-pleated sheets" and "alpha-helices". The further folding of a protein that gives it its own unique overall structure is its tertiary structure. The tertiary structure of a protein is determine and also stabilized by chemical interactions such as hydrogen bonds, ionic bonds, Van der Waals forces and hydrophobic interactions. Further, many proteins form multisubunit complexes, and the way these interact identifies the quaternary structure of the protein.

The following sections outline common methods that are used to monitor proteins, analyze their composition and mass, and determine subunit structure in biomedicine. They also outline various methods used to determine secondary, tertiary and quaternary structures of proteins, and identify various post-translational modifications.

B. Basic methods for protein analysis

Determination of protein content

Three methods are commonly used to quantify proteins in biological samples. Two of these are colorimetric assays named after their inventors, Lowry, who developed the first simple method for protein quantitation in 1951 (1), and Bradford (2), who developed a more sensitive colorimetric assay in 1976. The fact that Lowry's paper is one of the most frequently cited papers in history attests to the importance of methods to monitor protein concentration.

The Bradford assay is commonly used today due to its sensitivity and simplicity. It is based on the ability of Coomassie Brilliant blue dye, which was first used to dye wool, to bind to proteins at acid pH. Binding leads to a color change, which provides a measure of the amount of total protein present. The binding of Coomassie Blue is nonspecific and irreversible. Most Bradford assays today are quantitated using automated plate readers at an OD of 595 nm. The amount of protein can be quantitated by comparing the absorbance with a standard curve prepared using a purified protein such as albumin.

While the Bradford assay is easy to carry out and relatively quantitative, the most accurate measure of protein concentration is using a spectrophotometric approach. This is based on the absorbance of ultraviolet light at 280 nm by the protein. The side chains of the amino acids tryptophan and tyrosine are primarily responsible for the absorbance, with a minor contribution of cystines (disulfide bonds). If the amino acid composition of the protein is known, the most accurate determination of protein concentration can be obtained with this method.

Gels and gradients for separation of macromolecules

The size of biomolecules such as proteins or a piece of DNA can be determined by separation on gradients or gels. For gradient separation, sucrose density gradients are frequently used. The gradient forms in a tube when the sucrose mixture is subjected to a high centrifugal force using an ultracentrifuge. The larger macromolecules migrate farther in the gradient, while smaller ones migrate less, giving a degree of separation that varies given the differences in size of the macromolecules being separated, the concentration of the sucrose in the gradient, and the complexity of the starting material. One of the major advantages of sucrose gradient separation is that it does not denature the proteins and thus, non-covalently bound proteins can be isolated as protein-protein complexes. The development of the ultracentrifuge in the early twentieth century, and their use to determine precise molecular weights, was a major advance in protein chemistry. For his efforts in the development and use of the ultracentrifuge, Theodor Svedberg won the Nobel Prize in Physics in 1926. Nevertheless, the ultracentrifuge did not become a standard tool for separating biomolecules until the late 1940s and later. Today, ultracentrifuges are manufactured that can generate speeds of 100,000 to 130,000 rpm (revolutions per minute) and g forces (measured against the force of gravity) of 600,000 $\times$ g to 1,000,000 $\times$ g, reducing the time required for centrifugation.

Sedimentation equilibrium

Sedimentation equilibrium is a method for measuring protein molecular masses in solution and for studying protein-protein interactions. It can be used to determine if the native state of a protein is multimeric (dimer, trimer, *etc.*), and determine the stoichiometry of complexes that form from two or more different proteins. Using an analytical ultracentrifuge (which allows the distribution of a protein to be measured while the sample is being centrifuged), its molecular mass can be calculated (independent of the shape of the molecule) with accuracy, usually within one or two percent.

Sucrose density gradients

Sucrose density gradients formed in an ultracentrifuge can be used to resolve proteins of different sizes in cell lysates or to resolve different polymeric forms of a molecule that are produced, for example, during the synthesis and assembly of the molecule in the cell. This provides important insights into the biosynthetic intermediates during the synthesis of complex multimeric proteins. Because sucrose density gradients are non-denaturing, they will resolve polymeric proteins whether they are covalently or non-covalently associated. They are therefore very useful as one means of identifying interacting proteins (see protein-protein interactions below).

Sedimentation velocity

Sedimentation velocity is a common application of gradients. It measures the rate at which macromolecules move in response to centrifugal force. The rate of sedimentation provides information about the molecular mass and the shape of the molecule. Velocity sedimentation experiments are carried out at high centrifugal force for short periods of time, usually only a few hours. Under the conditions used, all macromolecules will "pellet" if centrifuged for longer periods of time.

Subcellular fractionation

The use of the ultracentrifuge and gradient separation techniques is not only applied to the study of proteins, but is also widely applied to subcelluiar fractionation studies, in which different cellular compartments (endosomes, lysosomes, mitochondria, endoplasmic reticulum, etc.) are resolved. These can be separated by methods that resolve according to size (velocity sedimentation) or density (density gradient separation). While sucrose gradients are often used for these studies, synthetic high density polymers such as Percoll and Nycodenz are now more widely. This is a useful tool, in conjunction with microscopy, to identify the subcelluiar compartments in which proteins reside.

Percoll is also used to separate different types of white blood cells based on their distinct densities.

Electrophoresis

Electrophoresis is a method used to separate macromolecules from complex mixtures by application of an electric field. The macromolecules are placed at one end of a matrix (referred to as a "gel") and are then subjected to the electrical current. Different macromolecules in the mixture will migrate at different speeds, depending on the nature of the gel and the characteristics of the macromolecules. Electrophoretic techniques can be applied to the separation of any macromolecule, including nucleic acids (DNA and RNA), proteins and carbohydrates. However, the principles of the separation and the matrices used may differ depending on the molecules that need to be separated. The electrophoretic separation of macromolecules in gels gives superior resolution to gradient separation techniques. The development of electrophoretic separation techniques was a major advance in the ability to resolve and characterize proteins and nucleic acids. For his efforts in development of electrophoresis as a method to separate proteins from complex mixtures, Arne Tiselius won the Nobel Prize in Chemistry in 1948.

Polyacrylamide gel electrophoresis (PAGE)

The use of PAGE gels have had a major impact on our ability to resolve proteins in complex mixtures, estimate their size, and determine some of their properties, it is one of the standard methods in biomedicine, in part because PAGE geis are so versatile. The development of PAGE gels, particular denaturing PAGE gels, has its roots in protein biochemistry. Two of the early pioneers in the development of modern electrophoretic separation techniques, F.W. Studier and J.V. Maizel, Jr., recently recounted the development of slab gels and SDS-PAGE technology in brief reviews in **Trends in Biochemical Sciences** (3,4).

Polyacrylamide gels are formed by the chemical cross-linking of acrylamide (the chemical monomer) with the chemical agent N,N'-methylene bisacrylamide (typically called "bis-acrylamide"). The polymerization reaction proceeds as a free-radical catalysis and is initiated by ammonium persulphate and the base TEMED (N,N,N',N'-tetramethylenediamine). More chemistry than you wanted? The bottom line: PAGE gels are remarkably versatile for performing high resolution separation of proteins and nucleic acids (such as for resolving DNA ladders in DNA sequencing reactions, or for RNase protection assays). In the case of proteins, PAGE gels can be used to separate them according to their size or charge, depending on other features of the gel matrix.

PAGE gels can be formed in tubes or as vertical "slab" gels, which are formed and run between two glass plates. PAGE gels are referred to by the percentage of acrylamide in the gels (4% PAGE gel, 10% PAGE gel, *etc.*). The percent acrylamide is varied depending on the nature and size of the macromolecule being separated and the method of separation used. In general, lower percentage gels are used for resolving nucleic acids or for isoelectric focusing, in which proteins are separated based on charge characteristics. Higher percentage gels (10% or greater) are normally used for separating proteins in SDS-PAGE.

SDS-PAGE

SDS (sodium dodecyl sulfate, also known as sodium lauryl sulfate)-PAGE is one of the most widely used methods for analyzing proteins. It is quantitative and separates proteins according to their size. Therefore, SDS-PAGE is widely used to determine the molecular mass of proteins (although it is inaccurate in some cases), to monitor protein purity, and, in conjunction with western blot analysis, to identify the presence of proteins in complex mixtures, to name but a few of the many uses of this technique. The development of the discontinuous buffer systems by Laemmli in 1970 (5) that are still used today greatly improved the resolution and reproducibility of SDS gels, and is generally credited with its popularity.

The power of the SDS-PAGE system relies not only on the gel but on the denaturing property of SDS. SDS is a negatively charged (anionic) detergent (you find it in some soaps and shampoos). When protein mixtures are boiled in SDS-containing buffers, they denature (unfold and assume a more linear configuration). The SDS binds to the denatured proteins quantitatively: the number of SDS molecules bound is proportional to the number of amino acids in the protein. The proteins thus have an overall negative charge, irrespective of their native charge. When proteins are denatured in SDS and subjected to PAGE, their mobility is inversely proportional to the log of their molecular weight, a property first reported in 1965 (6). Thus, large proteins migrate slower, whereas the smaller proteins migrate more quickly and move further into the gel.

Most SDS-PAGE gels are prepared with a narrow "stacking gel" above the primary separating gel. The stacking gel is a low percentage polyacrylamide; when the proteins migrate through the stacking gel and hit the resolving gel, it creates what has been referred to as a "traffic jam", such that all the proteins enter the resolving gel at essentially the same time, improving resolution and reproducibility.

Reducing and non-reducing SDS-PAGE

Most SDS-PAGE gels are run under reducing conditions, meaning that agents that reduce disulfide bonds, such as 2-mercaptoethanol (2-ME), are incorporated into the SDS-containing loading buffers. The presence of 2-ME serves two functions. First, it reduces the covalent bonds that might exist between muitimeric protein complexes. Second, it reduces covalent bonds that exist within a protein so that it achieves a more extended structure when boiled in SDS, which improves resolution and permits more accurate estimates of its molecular mass. Under non-reducing conditions, proteins can migrate aberrantly on SDS-PAGE gels. However, the comparison of isolated proteins on reducing and non-reducing SDS-PAGE (such as when coupled with immunoprecipitation using specific antibodies) provides an easy way to determine if a protein of interest might be covalently associated with another protein within a cell.

Native (non-denaturing) PAGE gels

Although SDS-PAGE is the most commonly used system for analyzing proteins, it does have some drawbacks. First, because of the denaturing activity of the SDS, it is often impossible to recover proteins in functional form, for example to measure enzymatic activity, once they have been fractionated on SDS-PAGE. In addition, important non-covalent protein-protein interactions are disrupted by SDS. Native gels offer advantages for both of these purposes. Native PAGE gels lack SDS. As a result, proteins migrate according to their own intrinsic charge (due to charged amino acids or post-translational modifications) as well as the sieving properties of the gel. In other words, they migrate very differently than on SDS-PAGE. Often, proteins can migrate as non-covalent complexes on these gels. Native gels in tubes can be used as a first separation for 2-dimensional gel electrophoresis, where complexes are separated in the first dimension in native gels, and then in the second by reducing SDS-PAGE. This helps in determining the nature of stable, non-covalent complexes (see below).

Isoelectric focusing (IEF)

Isoelectric focusing gels separate proteins according to their isoelectric points (pI). The pI of a protein is defined as the pH at which it has no net charge; below that pH, the protein has a net positive charge, while above it the protein is negatively charged. Isoelectric focusing gels are capable of high resolution, separating proteins with pIs that differ by less than 0.1 pH units. The "gel" component of IEF gels is usually polyacrylamide, although agarose can be used. The separation is achieved by introduction of "ampholytes", which are synthetic compounds of differing pHs. When subjected to an electric current, they form a pH gradient. Proteins will migrate toward that position at which they have no net charge (the "zwitterions" form), which reflects their isoelectric point.

IEF is an especially useful system for analyzing the microheterogeneity of proteins, such as revealing differences in glycosylation status, or identifying different phospho-isoforms. Frequently, these differences are not revealed on SDS-PAGE but are readily evident on IEF.

Two-dimensional (2D) gel electrophoresis

2D gel electrophoresis is a way to couple different gel systems with different resolving powers to dramatically improve separations and resolution of complex mixtures of proteins. 2D gel electrophoresis is an incredibly useful analytic pool, and provides a foundation for what is now referred to as "proteomics". The two most common types of 2D gel combine the power of IEF with SDS-PAGE, or combines non-reducing with reducing SDS-PAGE. In the first combination, proteins are separated in tubes by IEF, and the first gel is then treated so that the proteins can migrate out of the gel. This gel is placed at the top of the second gel and subjected to the next separation technique (SDS-PAGE). This allows for fine detail mapping of protein composition of cells (or subcellular organelles). If the proteins have come from cells that have been metabolically labeled with radioactive precursors, they can be directly visualized on film. Alternatively, 2D gels can be silver stained to reveal differences in protein composition of cells (or subcellular organelles) at different stages of development, or upon treatment with a drug, or even to monitor changes in protein expression during an infection with bacteria or viruses. This may involve what is euphemistically called the stare and compare approach, where long hours are spent looking for differences between two gels. More recently, computer programs that help overlay 2 different gels and identify differences between them have been developed to help expedite analysis. The identity of the proteins that change in expression can then be identified by candidate antibodies (by western blotting) or by sequencing using mass spectroscopy.

Two-dimensional non-reducing/reducing gels are processed similarly. The protein mixtures (for example, extracts from cells that have been metabolically labeled) are fractionated first under non-reducing and non-denaturing conditions. The gel is turned on its side and the proteins resolved in the first dimension are then denatured and resolved in the

Figure 1. Two-dimensional polyacrylamide gel electrophoresis

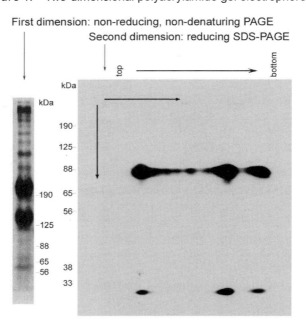

second dimension under reducing conditions. Figure 1 shows cell extracts from metabolically-labeled plasma cells (which synthesize and secrete antibodies; see Chapter 4) that have been fractionated on native gels in the first dimension, and then resolved in the second dimension under denaturing and reducing SDS-PAGE gels. The antibody produced by this cell is IgM which has many intracellular oligomeric forms as shown in the native gel in the first dimension, and these can approach sizes estimated to be 1 million Daltons. Using a reducing SDS-PAGE second dimension, each of the oligomeric species can be shown to be comprised of a typical IgM heavy chain, which is about 85,000 Daltons (or 85 kiloDaltons, or kDa) and a light chain, estimated to be 23 kDa. Molecular weight estimates are made by running "markers" of known molecular weight in each gel. Chapter 4 provides more information on the structure of antibodies and their function.

Detection of proteins in gels

It's great to be able to fractionate proteins in gels, but how do you see them once the fractionation is completed? There are a number of ways to detect proteins in gels. One of a number of stains can be used to reveal their presence, autoradiography (exposure to photographic film) can be used if the proteins have been metabolically labeled or had a radioactive tag added, or they can be identified by immunoblotting (also called western blotting).

Identification of proteins in gels by staining

A number of reagents can be used to nonspecifically or selectively stain proteins, thus allowing the visualization of protein bands or spots in gels.

Coomassie brilliant blue

Coomassie blue is a common dye used for protein chemistry because of its ability to bind to proteins, as well as other substances. Proteins are stained in the PAGE gel following treatment of the gel with a methanol/acetic acid solution, which causes the proteins in the individual bands to precipitate. Coomassie blue staining is not highly sensitive: the detection limit is about 0.3 to 1 µg protein in a band. However, for many screening purposes, Coomassie blue dyes are adequate to reveal the complexity and abundance of proteins in gels.

Ponceau S (Ponceau red)

Ponceau red differs from Coomassie blue staining in that it can be used to stain proteins after transfer to a membrane, and provides a rapid way to "visually" quantitate proteins on the membrane. Staining with Ponceau red is reversible, and the proteins can then be characterized by Western blotting (see below) following destaining of the membrane. Ponceau red is 1 to 2 orders of magnitude more sensitive than Coomassie blue.

Silver staining

Silver can be used to stain proteins because of the ability of silver to bind to chemical sidechains in the amino acids, including carboxyl and sulfhydryl groups. Silver staining has a much greater sensitivity than Coomassie or Ponceau staining, and can detect as little as 2 ng protein. It is commonly used to stain proteins separated by 2-dimensional electrophoresis since the small amount of material recovered in the second dimension, especially when IEF and SDS-PAGE are combined, can often not be detected by other, less sensitive methods. Because silver staining is irreversible, it sometimes creates problems when these spots are sequenced or otherwise characterized by mass spectroscopy.

Zinc staining

Zinc (or copper) is sometimes used for staining because staining with these metals represent "negative" staining protocols for SDS-PAGE. The polyacrylamide in the gel is stained but SDS, which coats the proteins, is not stained, thus excluding the metal from the protein bands. Zinc staining is more sensitive than Ponceau but less sensitive than Silver staining. Importantly, the proteins can be transferred and analyzed after the staining procedure.

Identification of proteins in gels using metabolic labeling

Metabolic labeling is a method in which the proteins in cells are labeled using radioactive forms of amino acids during their synthesis in the cell. Metabolic labeling is used to examine the different steady state pools of proteins within cells. The most common amino acid precursors are ^{35}S-labeled mixtures of methionine and cysteine. Proteins can also be labeled using precursors that are incorporated into post-translational modifications, such as phosphate groups or sugars incorporated into carbohydrates such as the N-linked glycans. The proteins can then be revealed within the gels by exposure to highly sensitive photographic film, a process known as autoradiography, or by phosphorimaging. Phosphorimaging is a technique in which radioactive decay is stored on phosphor screens, which can then be read by laser imaging into a computer. Phosphorimaging is more sensitive and has a greater dynamic range than film. Phosphorimaging can be used for quantitating ^{35}S or ^{125}I, but not tritium (^{3}H) or ^{14}C.

Pulse chase analysis

Most metabolic labeling studies use labeling periods of one to a few hours in an attempt to label the entire pool of a particular protein (or proteins) being synthesized by a cell. Pulse-chase analysis is a specialize form of metabolic labeling in which radioactive amino acids are added for very short periods of time, usually for a few minutes (the "pulse"), washed away, and then the cells are exposed only to nonradioactive forms of the same amino acids (in excess). The cells are then harvested and the proteins extracted for study. Pulse-chase analysis is used to study protein synthesis and processing, to examine the intracellular localization of nascent (newly synthesized) proteins over time, to examine their secretion, or monitor their degradation.

Western blot analysis (Immunoblotting)

Western blotting is a technique analogous to Southern and Northern blotting (see Chapter 2), but for proteins. The method was first reported in 1979 (7), following the description of the successful transfer procedure for DNA developed by E.M. Southern. Since Southern blotting was the first blotting method developed, the technique is presented in more detail in that section. After fractionating proteins on polyacrylamide gels, the proteins can be transferred quantitatively to membranes by capillary action or by electroblotting. Capillary transfer is lengthy and highly inefficient (10–20% of the proteins transfer), whereas electroblotting is rapid (2 to 3 hr) and efficient. In electroblotting, a membrane is placed next to a gel and submerged in a buffer. An electric current is passed at right angels to the gel, and the proteins are transferred onto the membrane.

The proteins that have been transferred to the membrane are then detected by a probe, an agent that can selectively and specifically identify a particular protein or related proteins. For western blot analysis, antibodies are the most common probes. The antibodies are directly labeled with a radioactive molecule, such as ^{125}I, so that its binding is detectable by autoradiography. Alternatively, it can be labeled with an enzyme, such as horseradish peroxidase (HRP) or alkaline phosphatase (AP). The blot can then be treated with the appropriate substrate solution, which is converted into an insoluble material which identifies the location of the antibody bound to the protein of interest on the membrane. However, most laboratories now use enhanced chemiluminescence (ECL) to detect the enzyme linked antibody (see Chapter 4).

There are a number of variations of the basic western blotting procedure described above. One of the most common is to take advantage of secondary antibodies. Secondary antibodies are "antibodies against antibodies" that have been labeled with ^{125}I or an enzyme. The use of secondary reagents negates the need to label primary antibodies. In this way, only a small number of secondary antibodies need to be labeled, rather than all of the primary antibodies of interest. Alternatively, biotinylated primary antibodies can be used. Biotin is a small molecular weight vitamin that is strongly bound by avidin, a protein from egg, which can be used as a secondary reagent rather than another antibody. This system is discussed further in Chapter 4.

Chromatography

Chromatography is a generic term that applies to a variety of methods that separate macromolecules. Chromatography is a method that takes advantage of columns (vertical tubes) that contain a matrix that is designed to trap or retard the passing of macromolecules based on a particular property such as size, charge, or composition. It is commonly used in protein purification. The mixture to be separated is added to the column and is flushed through by adding volumes of a buffer designed for the column. Flow is achieved by gravity or small pumps, although specialized equipment can also be used (see HPLC and FPLC below). Material flowing through the column is collected in tubes by automated fraction collectors for further analysis. The most common forms of chromatography are summarized below.

Gel filtration (or "size exclusion") chromatography

Gel filtration chromatography is based on a sieving method in which proteins are separated on the base of their size. Usually, columns are packed with a porous gel. The pores in the gel, which are essentially small holes, allow molecules of a predefined size or smaller to enter the pores, whereas the larger molecules are excluded. These larger molecules flow quickly through the gel and exit the column first, while the smaller molecules flow more slowly. Therefore, larger volumes of liquid are required to flush the smaller molecules out of the gel. In general, the volume required is inversely proportional to the size of the molecule. Unlike other methods of column chromatography, gel filtration chromatography is a method in which all proteins are expected to flow through the column and are separated based on the speed at which they exit. All other chromatographic techniques are based on retention of proteins by one or more properties.

Common media for gel filtration columns include agarose-based beads, such as Sepharose and Superose, cellulose based beads, and composites (agarose and dextran = Superdex; dextran and acrylamide beads = Sephacryl).

Ion exchange chromatography

Ion exchange chromatography is a method used to isolate proteins based on their charge. Both anion exchange columns (positively charged columns that are used to isolate negatively charged proteins) and cation exchange columns (negatively charged columns to isolate positively charged molecules) are available. Proteins that are bound to ion exchange columns are generally released or "desorbed" by increasing the salt concentration, which is often accomplished using a salt gradient. The higher the charge of the protein, the higher the salt concentration required to desorb it. Alternatively, altering the pH of the buffers can be used to desorb the bound proteins.

There are a number of ion exchange resins commonly used including anionic cellulose or dextran resins like DEAE-cellulose or DEAE-Sephadex, respectively, and cationic resins including CM-cellulose and CM-Sephadex.

Adsorption and partitioning matrices

Adsorption and portioning matrices retard the flow of a protein based on its physical characteristics. There are a large number of gels that function in this capacity. One example is hydrophobic interaction chromatography, which is a method used to enrich proteins that have significant hydrophobic groups. These columns generally are hydrophilic in nature. Most columns used in hydrophobic chromatography include a phenyl agarose matrix system. Common matrices include Phenyl-Sepharose and octyl-sepharose gels.

Affinity chromatography

Affinity chromatography is a method to specifically isolate a protein based on one of two methods. The most common form of affinity chromatography is an antibody based method in which antibodies that are specific for a particular protein are covalently coupled to a column matrix, often some form of Sepharose activated by an agent such as cyanogen-bromide. Material containing the antigen of interest, such as extracts of cells in which recombinant proteins have been expressed or supernatants from cultures in which proteins have been secreted during tissue culture, are passed over the columns. Only those proteins for which the antibodies are specific will bind to these columns. After washing, they can then be eluted with at low pH (2.5–3.5) or using chaotropic salts. Chaotropic salts (such as sodium thiocyanate or ammonium sulfate), like low pH, disrupt antigen-antibody and protein-protein interactions, allowing the bound material on the column to be eluted. Affinity chromatography is frequently used in purifying recombinant proteins because it gives one of the highest degrees of purity in a single step of any chromatographic method.

In addition to the use of antibodies, other agents are used for affinity chromatography. For example stretches of 6 histidine residues (introduced by recombinant DNA technology at the N or C terminus of a protein) bind to nickel. Therefore, nickel columns are used to purify his-tagged recombinant proteins. Protein A and protein G are frequently used to purify antibodies (see Chapter 4) In addition, lectins, which are proteins that recognize specific carbohydrate moieties, are frequently used to purify glycoproteins by affinity chromatography. Lectins can also be used as probe alternatives to antibodies for western blotting. Common lectins used for these studies include concanavalin A, a lectin isolated from jack beans which binds mannose residues, and ricin, a lectin from castor beans which binds galactose residues. Ricin is extremely toxic, so much so that it is considered a prime bioterrorist weapon.

High-performance liquid chromatography (HPLC)

HPLC is a generic term that refers to chromatography using fully automated equipment and "high performance" adsorbents for isolating and purifying compounds. The most common form of HPLC is reversed phase HPLC (RP-HPLC), which has very high resolving power for peptides and proteins up to 100 kiloDaltons (kDa), although it is best used for proteins of 30 kDa and smaller. It is based on the use of hydrophobic "reversed-phase" surfaces (usually silica with hydrophobic chains) that interact with the polypeptides or proteins added to the column. When the organic component of the mobile phase reaches a critical concentration, defined by the properties of the polypeptide, it is eluted in a very sharp peak. RP-HPLC can be used to distinguish between variants of hormones such as insulin that differ by a single amino acid. Given its high resolving power, it is the method of choice to purify proteins before subjecting them to Mass Spectroscopy.

RP-HPLC can, however, cause some transient denaturation during the adsorption and elution procedure, and therefore care must be taken if the investigator desires fully functional proteins. It is therefore mostly used to separate small molecules and polypeptides.

Fast protein liquid chromatography (FPLC)

FPLC is a high performance system that was designed for protein fractionation by the company Amersham Pharmacia Biotech. FPLC uses all of the standard protein separation methods including gel filtration, ion exchange chromatography, affinity chromatography, *etc*. FPLC is designed to improve the speed and resolution when separating proteins.

Dialysis and ultrafiltration

Once proteins have been isolated by column chromatography, they frequently need to be stored in a new buffer or concentrated for further use. To change the buffer, the mixture containing the protein is placed in dialysis tubing, which is a semipermeable tubing that allows small molecules and water to be exchanged between the contents within the tube and the outside of the tube. By "dialyzing" the material against several changes of the desired buffer, the buffer within the dialysis tubing will be replaced by the buffer outside of the tube by coming into equilibrium with the outside buffer. The dialysis tubing can have various exclusion sizes, such that small molecules below a particular molecular weight cutoff (1,000 Da, 10,000 Da, *etc.*) can also be dialyzed out of the protein mix.

Ultrafiltration is a process by which the volume in which macromolecules have been obtained can be concentrated. Ultrafiltration can be done under pressure or using centrifugal force. The material to be concentrated is applied in the upper chamber above a filter with the desired molecular weight exclusion so that the protein of interest does not go through the filter but other small molecules and buffer do. Proteins mixtures can be concentrated 10 to 100-foid or more using this method.

C. Characterization of primary, secondary, tertiary and quaternary structures of proteins

Protein sequencing (primary protein structure)

Three different methods were initially developed for direct sequencing of proteins, These included the Sanger, Dansyl chloride, and Edman degradation techniques. All three were laborious, required huge amounts of starting material (grams or more), and also required long periods of time, often years, to complete the sequence of a short protein. For the development of one of the methods of protein sequencing and using it to solve the sequence and structure of insulin, Frederick Sanger received the first of his two Nobel Prizes in Chemistry in 1958. He was to receive his second in 1980 for developing what became the most widely used method for sequencing DNA.

The ability to indirectly deduce the sequence of a protein has come a long ways since the 1950s and 1960s, and these original methods are only rarely used today. The most common ways to sequence proteins now is to clone its corresponding cDNA or genomic sequence and deduce the amino acid sequence from the nucleotide sequence. Using this method, the genomes of entire species, including man, have been obtained in a relatively short period of time (see Chapter 2). In addition, mass spectroscopy is now commonly employed to aid in the identification and sequencing of proteins.

Mass Spectrometry (MS)

A mass spectrometer is an instrument that can determine the mass of molecules that have been ionized (electrically charged). MS has become a key tool in proteomics research because it can analyze and identify compounds that are present at extremely low concentrations (as little as 1 pg) in very complex mixtures by analyzing its unique signature.

There are three parts to a mass spectrometer: the ion source, the mass analyzer, and the detector. Three broad types of ionization methods are used in MS, including electrospray ionization, electron ionization, and matrix-assisted laser desorption/ionization. Analyzers use dispersion or filtering methods to collect and sort ions according to their mass-to-charge ratios. Several types of analyzers exist, including quadrupole mass analyzers, quadrupole ion trap mass analyzers, fourier-transform MS analyzers, and time-of-flight mass analyzers, to name but a few. The ions are then detected by various light or charge detectors. Frequently, MS procedures are known by the combination of ionizer and analyzer that is used. For example, matrix-assisted laser desorption/ionization (MALDI) MS, combined with a time-of-flight (TOF) analyzer is referred to as MALDI-TOF MS. A critical concern in MS is that the methods used for ionization can be so harsh that they may generate very little product to measure at the end. The development of "soft" desorption ionization methods by John Fenn and Koichi Tanaka, which allowed the application of MS to biomolecules on a wide scale, earned them a share of the Nobel Prize in Chemistry in 2002.

MS is used following 2-dimensional gel protein separation for proteomic analysis. It can be used to rapidly and unequivocally identify the protein in a spot on a 2-dimensional gel, even at low abundance. Mass mapping is used to identify a protein by cleaving it into short peptides. The mass spectrometer can then be used to deduce the protein's identity by matching the observed peptide masses (which are determined with incredible accuracy) with protein databases. MS has therefore become a prime method for helping to understand changes in the expression of proteins in cells during lineage development, in infected cells versus their normal counterparts, or in transformed cells. While methods to examine differentially expressed genes have also been developed (see Chapter 3), the expression of mRNA does not always mean that the concomitant protein is expressed, and thus approaches that allow for direct protein identification are important. In addition to identifying proteins, tandem MS can be used to directly sequence peptides from proteins by colliding them with non reactive gas and analyzing the fragmented ions that are produced. Not only does this provide direct amino acid sequence information, but also reveals post-translational modifications such as phosphorylation, sulfination, and the size, complexity can dramatically change the function of a protein. Therefore, proteomic analysis is an indispensable addition to genomic analysis.

Methods to determine secondary and tertiary protein structure

While MS is now widely used to determine partial sequences of proteins for purposes of proteomic analysis, it does not proved information about the secondary or three-dimensional structure of protein. Methods that are commonly employed for these purposes are circular dichroism for secondary structure analysis and x-ray diffraction and nuclear magnetic resonance (NMR) for obtaining 3-dimenstional structures of proteins. X-ray diffraction and NMR are frequently considered complementary techniques. The importance of both x-ray diffraction and NMR for the structural analysis of proteins cannot be underestimated: the development and use of these methods have led to several Nobel Prized (seeTable1).

Circular dichroism (CD) spectroscopy

Circular dichroism is a method that provides basic information on the overall secondary structure of a protein, including the percentage of beta sheets and alpha helices. Random coil structures also generate characteristic CD spectra. CD spectroscopy measures differences in the absorption of left-and right-handed polarized light that arises from asymmetric structures. Secondary structural analyses are usually carried out in the "far-uv" spectrum (190–250 nm). Using CD spectroscopy in the "near-uv" spectrum (250–350 nm) can sometimes provide some information on the tertiary structure of the protein. CD spectroscopy is also used to measure structural changes that might occur upon the interaction of two proteins, or upon receptor-ligand interactions.

X-ray crystallography

X-ray crystallography was the first method developed for determining the 3-dimensional structure of a protein and remains the method of choice for solving the structure of proteins that can be crystallized. X-ray crystallography has also been used to elucidate the structure of multi-protein complexes and protein-DNA complexes. The method is based on principles established over ninety years ago, and referred to a as Bragg's Law. The Braggs (a father and son "dynamic duo"), shared the Nobel Prize in Physics in 1915 for their work demonstrating that x-rays could be used for structural analysis, a year after Max von Laue receive the Nobel Prize for demonstrating that crystals diffracted x-rays. Bragg's law (without going into the physics) allows information about a crystal structure to be obtained from x-ray diffraction data. The diffraction peaks can be used to reconstruct an electron density map, which is accomplished by Fourier transforming the diffraction intensities. Obviously, analysis of x-ray diffraction data is a computationally intense exercise!

X-ray crystallography is only useful if crystals can be grown from purified proteins. This is because the presence of precise, repeating structure present in crystals is essential for using x-ray diffraction to solve 3-dimenstional structures. For this reason, the structure of many intact proteins cannot be accomplished using x-ray diffraction. Consequently, a "divide and conquer" approach is often used, in which protein are expressed as individual domains for structural analysis. A protein domain is typically defined as an independent folding unit within an overall protein structure. Thus, proteins can be broken down into their component parts. Individual domains of interest, such as regions that contain catalytic sites of enzymes or protein interaction domains, are crystallized and the structure of these domains independently solved.

The resolution of the structure obtained with x-ray diffraction is highly dependent on the quality of the crystals that can be grown, Better crystals can usually be produced with smaller molecules (or protein domains) than with larger molecules. The structural resolution is defined in terms of angstroms (Å): for example, the crystal structure of protein X at 2.4 Å, or 1.8 Å, *etc*. An Å is 0.1 nanometer, or 10^{-10} meter. At 2 Å resolution, peptides can distinguished in a protein, but resolutions of 1.5 Å or better are required to distinguish individual atoms, which allows much more precise understanding of the molecule. An clear understanding of the 3-dimensional structure of a protein (or protein domains) is crucial for a variety of studies, including mapping contact sites between an enzyme and its substrate, delineating the nature of antigen binding sites in antibodies or identifying potential target sites for therapeutics in the treatment of viral infections. High resolution structural analysis is also important for helping design agonistic or antagonistic ligands for receptors that function abnormally in disease, to name but a few of the many ways structural information has been useful.

Nuclear magnetic resonance (NMR) spectroscopy

For those proteins that cannot be crystallized, NMR is the method of choice for tertiary structural analysis. NMR was first developed in the 1940s but it wasn't until the 1970s and later that it could be applied to solving structures of biomolecules. While NMR is generally less sensitive than x-ray diffraction and data collection requires longer periods of time, recent advances have significantly improved NMR technology.

NMR requires high magnetic fields and radio-frequency pulses to alter the spin state of nuclei. These spin states differ depending on the environment the nuclei are in. Thus, the nature of nearby atoms and their distances influence the chemical shifts of the nuclei that can be observed by NMR. Only one naturally occurring atom in proteins, hydrogen (1H), can be observed by NMR. Therefore, proteins are usually uniformly labeled with the other atoms that can be observed by NMR, 13-carbon or 15-nitrogen.

Quaternary protein structure: Protein-protein interactions

Proteins do not always function alone, but frequently function as dimers, trimers, or higher order polymers of single proteins (homodimers, homotrimers, *etc.*) or more than one protein (heterodimers, heterotrimers, *etc.*). A number of methods have been developed to determine whether a protein exists in native form or as part of a higher order polymer within cells.

Non-reducing/non-denaturing gels and gradients

These are often used to isolate proteins from cellular extracts in their native states. The identities of the component chains can then be identified by resolving them on denaturing and reducing/denaturing gels to determine if proteins are non-covalently or covalently associated, as described in detail earlier in this chapter. This method works well if the identity of one or more of the interacting proteins is known, and is often combined with co-immunoprecipitation studies.

Co-immunoprecipitation

Co-immunoprecipitation uses antibodies to one component of a protien complex to immunoprecipitate it, causing the antibody-bound complex to fall out of solution. If the protein is stably bound to another protein, both interacting proteins will be immunoprecipitated by the antibody. Alternatively, protein A or protein G coupled to a solid support can be used to facilitate the isolation of the antibody-bound antigens (see Chapter 4 for more information). The immunoprecipitated material can be denatured in SDS and resolved on SDS-PAGE gels. Interacting proteins can then be identified by western blotting, if the identity of the interacting protein is suspected. If unknown proteins are suspected, other methods are often used. For example, the proteins can first be radioactively labeled by metabolic labeling so that the size, and other properties, of the other interacting components can be determined following immuno-precipitation using autoradiography. As in all studies of protein-protein interactions, artifacts can occur and additional studies to confirm that co-immunoprecipitated proteins indeed interact *in vivo* are always warranted.

Far western blot

The far western blot is a modification of the western blot designed to study protein-protein interactions. As in a western blot, proteins (usually from cell lysates) are first resolved on the gel of choice (reducing SDS-PAGE or native PAGE) and then transferred to a membrane. The prey proteins on the membrane are probed with a known protein of direct visualization, or identified using a secondary antibody. If the bait protein is bound to one or more proteins on the membrane, it will then be identifiable. Far western analysis can also be done "in-gel" by first renaturing the resolved prey proteins in the gel and then using the bait to probe the gel.

Pull-down assays

The pull-down technique has become a valuable tool to identify interacting proteins. It can be used to confirm previously suspected interactions suggested from results of co-immunoprecipitation studies, results from non-denaturing gels or density gradient analysis, *etc.* or used to as a screening assay to search for previously unknown interacting partners for a protein of interest. Pull-down assays require that one of the interacting partners, the bait, be available in purified form. This is usually accomplished using recombinant DNA techniques. In addition, the bait must be tagged in some way. It can be tagged with biotin (hence, biotin pull-down assays) or as a fusion protein with a sequence tag produced using prokaryotic or eukaryotic expression system (see Chapter 3). The bait is then used to interact with prey proteins obtained both the bait and its interacting partners. The interacting partners can then be resolved on SDS-PAGE and identified by staining the gel and/or western blotting, *etc.*

Cross-linking agents

While many proteins can be isolated by one of the methods described above, many functional protein interactions are only transient, making their identification difficult. This is where cross-linking reagents can be useful. These serve to covalently cross-linking proteins that are sufficiently close in space to be bridged by the cross-linker. This approach can work well to identify proteins can then be isolated from detergent lysates of the cells and analyzed. The cross-linking agents are frequently produced with a cleavable internal bond, such as a disulfide bond, so that the two interacting proteins can be separated from one another by reducing agents.

This approach can also be applied to proteins in cell lysates. In principal, the cross-linker is small enough to only span interacting molecules. However, in a concentrated cell lysate, many proteins might be "nearby" without being involved in functional interactions. To get around this problem, purified bait proteins that are pre-reacted with one end of a heterobifunctional cross-linked agents is often added to potential prey proteins in cell lysates and allowed to interact. For these studies, the other part of the bifunctional agent is not reactive until activated, usually by UV light. The interacting proteins are then analyzed to identify potential prey.

Yeast two-hybrid screen

This is a very powerful genetic approach that not only allows an investigator to determine if there are interacting partners for a known bait protein, but also provides a genetic clone of the prey for easy identification. Yeast two-hybrid screens are used for identifying a variety of interacting proteins, including those that are transcriptional activators. The beauty of the yeast two-hybrid system is that it can be used to identify not only stably interacting proteins, but also those proteins that associate only transiently in the cell.

The yeast two-hybrid system was first developed in 1989 (8) and uses a bait protein to screen for an interacting protein(s) from a cDNA library from the same species. Yeast (Saccharomyces cerevisiae) serves as a host for the cDNA library screen. The yeast contains 2 plasmids, one with the gene for the bait protein, and one that contains the cDNA library (representing all the potential prey proteins). The system is set up so that any protein that interacts with the bait will cause transcription of a reporter gene, thus giving a visual readout of transcription, and identifying a yeast clone that contains a cDNA that encodes a protein that interacts with the bait.

The bait and prey cDNAs are expressed as fusion proteins with two different protein domains that, when they interact, reconstitute a transcriptional activation protein that drives a reporter gene. The Gal4 transcription activation protein is the system of choice. Gal4 activates genes encoding enzymes that are required by the yeast for galactose utilization.

Gal4 is an 881 amino acid long protein that can be separated into a DNA binding domino (amino acids 1to 147) and an activation domain (amino acids 771 to 881). The bait is fused to the coding sequence of the DNA-binding domain, and individual clones from the cDNA library are fused to the transcriptional activating domain. When the two components of the transcription factor are brought together by the interaction of bait and prey proteins, it is reconstituted and the reporter gene, which is regulated by Gal4 cognate sequences, is expressed. This system can be used to identify interacting proteins from a variety of eukaryotic species that mediate a variety of functions, from signal transduction to transcription, and has been one of the most useful systems developed to identify interacting partners.

Fluorescence resonance energy transfer (FRET)

Fret is another powerful method for identifying proteins that interact within live cells. FRET depends on the ability to stably or transiently express each of two different interacting proteins in a cell that are labeled with fluorescent molecules that are capable of transferring energy. In general, the proteins to be studied using FRET are genetically modified as fusion proteins to contain one of two different green fluorescent protein derivatives (see Chapter 5 for more information). Because it is a microscopic method, FRET provides direct insights into the intracellular compartments in which protein-protein interactions occur.

Chapter 2

DETECTION AND ANALYSIS OF NUCLEIC ACIDS

A.   Introduction

The year 2003 marked the 50th anniversary of the paper by James Watson and Francis Crick reporting the solution of the three dimensional structure of deoxyribonucleic acid (DNA) (9). This achievement earned them a Nobel Prize, which they shared in 1962 with Maurice Wilkins for his crystallographic studies on DNA structure (Table 2). It also set the stage for a new era which led to breakthroughs in our understanding of the genetic code and the development of techniques that allowed for the rapid sequencing of DNA. Eventually, the entire genome of a number of organisms would be sequenced, culminating in the complete sequencing of the human genome in 1991. An understanding of DNA structure also permitted the development of methods to clone and manipulate DNA (recombinant DNA technology), as well as alter the sequence of DNA using site directed mutagenesis to gain insights into the function of individual proteins. The advent of the molecular biology revolution also allowed us to begin to understand how genes are regulated. The regulation of gene expression is not only the key to our understanding of how genes are turned on and off, but to how genes are regulated in a tissue specific manner, how cellular differentiation occurs, and how tissues and organs develop. From the development of simple methods to clone, sequence, and manipulate DNA came a realization of its power to help solve the genetic basis of human disease. This, in turn, resulted in the development and evolution of the Biotechnology Industry, an industry that was founded to develop ways to synthesize hormones, enzymes and other proteins, rather than rely on their purification from natural sources. The production of hormones in the laboratory made it practical to treat patients on a large scale for the first time.

The description of the "double helix" by Watson and Crick, while a watershed discovery, was not the beginning of our understanding of the

Table 2. Selected Nobel Laureates (Molecular Biology)

George W. Beadle Edward L. Tatum Joshua Lederberg	genetic recombination and discoveries on the chemical basis of genes in bacteria	1958[†]
Severo Ochoa Arthur Kornberg	synthesis of RNA and DNA	1959[†]
Francis H. C. Crick James D. Watson Maurice H. F. Wilkins	discovery of the 3-dimensional structure of DNA as a double helix; base pairing	1962[†]
François Jacob André Lwoff Jacques Monod	analysis of how genes are regulated (bacteria and viruses); advent of "molecular biology" era	1965[†]
Robert W. Holley Har Gobind Khorana Marshall W. Nirenberg	solution of the genetic code; chemistry of protein synthesis	1968[†]
Max Delbrück Alfred D. Hershey Salvador E. Luria	mechanisms of replication and genetic structure of viruses (bacteriophages)	1969[†]
David Baltimore Renato Dulbecco Howard M. Temin	characterization and function of RNA tumor viruses; the discovery of reverse transcriptase	1975[†]
Werner Arber Daniel Nathans Hamilton O. Smith	discovery of restriction enzymes; use of restriction enzymes for genetic analysis	1978[†]
Paul Berg Walter Gilbert Frederick Sanger	first recombinant DNA (Berg); DNA sequencing methods (Gilbert, Sanger)	1980[*]
Richard J. Roberts Phillip A. Sharp	"split genes" (intron/exon structure of eukaryotic genes)	1993[†]
Kary B. Mullis Michael Smith	invention of the PCR (Mullis); site-directed mutagenesis (Smith)	1993[*]

[†]Nobel Prize in Physiology or Medicine
[*]Nobel Prize in Chemistry

composition of DNA or its role in the makeup of genes. The idea that genes are independent and heritable is usually traced to the studies of the Czech monk, Gregor Mendel, who demonstrated that phenotypic traits are inherited in his studies of peas in 1866. Soon afterwards (1868), Friedrich Miescher isolated a new substance that was neither protein nor sugar from the nucleus of cells which he called nucleic acid. However, the link between nucleic acid and genetic makeup was not made until the landmark publication by Oswald Avery and his colleagues, Colin MacLeod and Maclyn McCarty, in 1944 (10). In this paper, they showed for the first time that hereditable traits could be transferred using purified

DNA from one bacterium to another (and its daughter cells). As is often true of ground-breaking discoveries, the acceptance of this one was tempered by skepticism due to the prevailing wisdom of the time that proteins were responsible for heredity. Indeed, the composition of the nucleic acids that made up the DNA was considered to be too simple to be responsible for something as complex as a gene. However, the conclusion from Avery's research was unmistakable: nucleic acids, and thus DNA, was responsible for the genetic makeup of an organism. How DNA was responsible for the transmission of genetic traits could only be understood after Watson and Crick had solved the 3-dimensional structure of DNA and the genetic code had been broken. But these ground-breaking studies would not have been possible without the work of Avery. While the awarding of a Nobel Prize is sometimes controversial (we'll come back to that later), the failure to award one to Avery has been considered by some to be one of the most egregious oversights in Nobel history.

Within 20 years of the discovery of the 3-dimensional structure of DNA, its chemical structure was solved, DNA replication was understood, and the basic parameters of how DNA is precisely transcribed into RNA (ribonucleic acid), which is then translated into protein, became clear. The development of many new technologies was required to achieve these breakthroughs, and many of the techniques that were invented for these discoveries remain in use today. Some of these were so instrumental in their applicability to solve biological problems that they also garnered Nobel Prizes for their inventors (Table 2).

The following are brief descriptions of some of the common methods used to manipulate nucleic acids, especially DNA.

B. Basic methods for nucleic acid analysis

Gels and gradients for separation of nucleic acids

The size of a piece of DNA, usually produced as the result of restriction digestion (see below) can be determined by separation on gradients or gels. For gradient separation, sucrose density gradients were common at one time but were supplanted by gels once electrophoretic separation techniques were developed. Two types of gel matrices are commonly used for the separation of nucleic acids: those made from polyacrylamide, and those using agarose. When a mixture of DNA fragments is applied to one end of the gel and subjected to an electric current, the DNA fragments migrate toward the positive pole of the field, the anode, due to the negatively charged phosphate groups that make up the DNA backbone. Following electrophoretic separation, the DNA can be visualized by one or more methods as discussed below.

Polyacrylamide gel electrophoresis (PAGE)

PAGE gels, as previously mentioned, are used for high resolution separation of nucleic acids, such as for resolving DNA ladders in DNA sequencing reactions or for RNase protection assays. For nucleic acid separation, PAGE gels served as the first matrix used to demonstrate that restriction fragments of nucleic acids could be resolved in gels, and their sizes could be calculated from their migration patterns (11). In general, relatively low percentage gels are used for resolving nucleic acids.

Agarose gel electrophoresis

Agarose gel electrophoresis is one of the standard methods of molecular biology and is a method used to resolve and separate nucleic acid fragments of different sizes. The use of agarose as a matrix to separate DNA was quickly adapted once it was established that DNA fragments could be separated by gel electrophoresis.

Agarose is a sugar polymer isolated from seaweed; when boiled and cooled, it forms a "gel", much like jello. The agarose gel serves to impede the migration of the DNA, so that larger fragments of DNA migrate slower than smaller fragments. Because DNA migrates in an electric field as a consequence of the phosphates on the DNA backbone, the charge to mass ratio is identical for all DNA fragments, irrespective of their length. As a result, while the separation is due to the charge of the DNA, the migration of DNA fragments is inversely proportional to the log (base 10) of the molecular weight of the fragment. Thus, if fragments of unknown size are compared with a control "ladder" containing fragments of known sizes (these are commercially available), the sizes of unknown fragments can be readily calculated. Depending on the concentration of agarose in the gels, DNA fragments from under 100 base pairs (bp) to 30,000 base pairs (30 kilobases, or kb) can be resolved by standard agarose gel electrophoresis. Following separation of the DNA, the fragments can be visualized in the gel using fluorescent dyes that intercalate (*i.e.*, insert) between the bases of the DNA helix. The most common dye used is ethidium bromide, which appears red upon exposure to ultraviolet light, but other dyes, such as SYBER green, are becoming increasingly popular.

Pulsed field electrophoresis

This is a method that allows for the separation of much larger fragments of DNA than standard agarose gel electrophoresis. In this method, the direction of the electrical current is altered periodically, allowing for the separation of fragments from 30 kb to several million base pairs.

Alkaline agarose gels

Agarose gel electrophoresis works well for separating double stranded DNA fragments and for the separation of RNA, but does not resolve single stranded DNA species. The incorporation of a base such as sodium hydroxide into the buffers used in the gels permits good resolution of single stranded DNAs.

Restriction enzymes and restriction fragments

Restriction endonucleases are enzymes that cleave DNA at specific sites. They are one of the most important tools in the analysis of DNA and for recombinant DNA technology. Restriction enzymes come from bacteria. They are a component of the "restriction-modification systems" of bacteria. These modification systems are thought to have evolved to help protect bacteria against foreign DNA, whether introduced by viral infection (by bacteriophages) or by DNA from other species of bacteria taken up by the host bacterium (see below). The fundamental work on restriction modification systems by Werner Arber, including the discovery of restriction enzymes, helped lead to the first insights into their sequence specificity by Kelly and Smith in 1970 (12) and to their use to characterize restriction fragments of viral DNA by Danna and Nathans in 1971 (11). These studies on restriction enzymes earned the Nobel Prize for Arber, Hamilton Smith and Daniel Nathans in 1978.

Hundreds of restriction enzymes (over 600 at this point) have been isolated. Restriction enzymes recognize short specific sequences in double stranded DNA. The sequences are generally palandromic, meaning they read the same (have the same nucleotides) in opposite orientations on the complementary DNA strands. Palandromic sequences can occur because of the base-pairing that is required in double stranded DNA (dsDNA). The 4 nucleotide bases adenine (A), cytosine (C), guanine (G) and thymine (T) exist in dsDNA as A-T and G-C complementary pairs. When the appropriate sequence is recognized, the restriction enzymes cut the DNA at specific sites within this recognition site, giving rise to a restriction fragment, which represents the piece(s) of DNA produced after cleaving the DNA with one or more restriction enzymes.

The actual cuts produced by a restriction enzyme can be "blunt" (that is, they cut at the same place on both strands of DNA) whereas others make symmetrical cuts with "overhangs". For example, the restriction enzyme *Eco*RI (isolated from the bacterium *Escherichia coli*) recognizes the DNA base sequence GAATTC and cuts between the G and A (on the opposite strand the sequence is CTTAAG, and the cut occurs between the A and G on that strand). Restriction enzymes are often classified by the number of nucleotides they recognize. Because *Eco*RI recognizes a 6 base pair sequence, it is called a "6-cutter". Most restriction enzymes recognize 4, 6 or 8 bp sequences, although some have longer recognition sites. The longer and more specific the sequence recognized by a restriction enzyme, the fewer of these sites that are expected to be present in any given stretch of DNA. While the majority of restriction enzymes recognize DNA sequences irrespective of their methylation status, some restriction enzymes recognize a sequence motif in unmethylated but not methylated DNA.

Restriction enzymes are a basic tool in the analysis of DNA (restriction mapping) and recombinant DNA technology. Restriction enzymes are used to enzymatically digest genomic DNA into fragments before electrophoretic separation and Southern blotting, to generate fragments of DNA for cloning into vectors, and production of small fragments from a gene for making probes for Southern or Northern blots. DNA can be digested to completion using restriction enzymes or, for the production of genomic libraries where large stretches of DNA are desired, partial digests can be carried out. Partial digestion means that the enzyme is used in sub-optimal concentrations and that the DNA is incubated with the enzyme for a limited period of time. In this way, large pieces of DNA with internal sites that have not been cut by the restriction enzyme are generated and can be used for cloning purposes.

Restriction fragment length polymorphism (RFLP)

RFLPs are a type of length polymorphism in the genomes of homologous segments of DNA of different individuals that have been digested with a restriction enzyme. The digested DNA is resolved on agarose gels, and specific probes are used to identify regions of the DNA that exhibit length polymorphisms. The use of RFLPs to help map genes involved in human diseases was first suggested by David Botstein (13), and is now widely used not only to help map genes that contribute to diseases, but in forensics for the precise identification of DNA samples (see below).

Single nucleotide polymorphisms (SNP)

SNPs are single base pair variations in the DNA sequence of an individual gene. They occur in the human population at a relatively high frequency and are very abundant, occurring at a rate of about 1 per 1000 base pairs. SNP genotypes are used in mapping disease susceptibility loci as well as in comparative genetics, evolutionary genetics, and forensic analysis.

Southern blotting

After resolving complex mixtures of DNA (such as restriction digested genomic DNA) on a gel, how can you determine which restriction fragment in a smear of DNA contains a particular gene? One method that was initially used was to manually cut slices out of the gel, isolate the DNA from the slices, and then hybridize the isolated DNA with a specific probe. This was not only highly laborious but also extremely inefficient. A second method, which revolutionized the ability to analyze DNA, was introduced by E.M. Southern in 1975 (14), and was rapidly adapted to the analysis of other macromolecules. Southern realized that because gels are porous, macromolecules within the gel could be transferred to another medium by a method called "blotting through". The mediums used are membranes, usually constructed of nitrocellulose or nylon. The DNA is denatured (with NaOH, since only ssDNA can transfer), the membrane is placed onto the gel, and then capillary action or a pump-based suction method is used to transfer the DNA from the gel onto the membrane using high salt solutions. While the capillary action method of transfer is "low tech", it is highly efficient and still used by many investigators since it takes longer and allows them the time to go home and sleep! The DNA is then immobilized on the membrane using heat (nitrocellulose) or ultraviolet light (nylon), and the entire membrane can now be probed.

Blotting methods work well for agarose gels but not for polyacrylamide gels, particularly the higher percentage gels used for proteins. For these, the transfer is accomplished by electroblotting (see Chapter 1).

Dot blotting and slot blotting

These are methods to immobilize bulk unfractionated DNA onto a membrane using a suction manifold. The manifolds have circular wells (dot blots) or slit wells (slot blots). They are frequently used to determine if a nucleic acid is present in a sample and to determine the relative abundance of the nucleic acid. They are most frequently used for RNA analysis. Since fractionation is not used, they do not rely on the integrity of the RNA. These blotting methods are now rarely used and have been supplanted almost entirely by polymerase chain reaction methods, which are more rapid, accurate, and quantitative.

Probes to identify nucleic acids on membranes

To identify a particular nucleic acid (whether DNA or RNA) on a membrane, probes are used. A probe is a general name for a substance that is used to specifically identify a macromolecule. It can be a chemical, an antibody, a protein, or a fragment of DNA.

For identifying nucleic acids on membranes, DNA probes are often used. These probes are labeled by one of several methods with either a radioactive isotope, a dye or fluorescent compound, or an enzyme. The probes are hybridized (annealed) to nucleic acids on the membrane. If a complementary nucleic acid is present, the probe anneals, and its presence can be detected by a method suited to the detection of the probe, depending on the labeling method. The probe must be single stranded in order to hybridize. As a result, labeled double stranded DNA fragments must be denatured prior to hybridization. Single stranded probes can also be synthesized using the appropriate vector (see below).

After hybridization reactions, membranes are washed in solutions containing formamide, SSC (a salt solution containing sodium chloride and sodium citrate) and SDS (sodium dodecyl sulfate). By reducing the concentration of SSC and increasing the temperature at which the membrane is washed, only highly complementary segments of nucleic acids will remain annealed to the probe. This is generally referred to as increasing the stringency between probe and target sequence.

Autoradiography (exposing the blot to x-ray film) is typically used to visualize the hybridization of a radioactive probe to the membrane. Alternatively, the hybridized probe can be identified and quantitated by phosphorimaging. For probes that have been labeled with fluorescent dyes or enzymes, colorimetric methods that rely on chemiluminescence can also be used (see Chapter 4).

C.   DNA sequencing

Introduction

DNA sequencing is, as the name implies, a method that reveals the linear sequence of nucleic acids within a stretch of DNA. DNA is composed of four nucleotide bases: adenine (A), cytosine (C), guanine (G), and thymine (T). The base present at a particular position in a DNA sequence is identified by the presence of a product of a chemical or enzymatic reaction in a gel. The ability to sequence DNA was a major advance for a number of reasons. First, it allows for the prediction of a potential open reading frame (ORF) for genes within a genomic DNA sequence. An ORF is the sequence that is transcribed and translated into protein, and in eukaryotic DNA is not contiguous but interrupted by intronic sequences. DNA sequencing is far more rapid and significantly cheaper than protein sequencing methods, and thus is the method of choice for most sequencing projects. The sequence of a protein can be used to predict its function by identifying potential protein interaction sites, DNA interaction sites, or motifs critical to enzymatic function or consensus enzyme recognition motifs. DNA sequencing also allows for the rapid identification of potential regulatory elements within genes (both upstream promoter sequences as well as intronic and 3′ enhancers) by comparing DNA sequence information with known transcription factor binding sites, or evaluating non-coding sequences in the introns around a gene that are conserved across species. These elements often predict sequences with regulatory functions. Sequencing therefore provides basic information about protein structure that can then be confirmed (or rejected) by directly testing these domains for functional activities.

Two major methods have been developed for the sequencing of DNA, one based on chemical methods (the "Maxam-Gilbert" method, named after its developers) and an enzymatic chain termination method often referred to as "dideoxy" sequencing or "Sanger sequencing" after its developer. Gilbert and Sanger shared with Nobel prize for these technical advances in 1980 with Paul Berg, who developed recombinant DNA techniques.

Both DNA sequencing techniques rely on reactions that generate oligonucleotide ladders, which terminate in definable nucleotides (A T G or C), although the methods used to achieve these are quite different. In both methods, a piece of DNA that can be manipulated in the sequencing reactions (often generated using restriction enzymes) is inserted into a cloning vector. Cloning vectors contain unique sites that flank both sides the cloned DNA fragment, the insert, to be sequenced. These sites are complementary to oligonucleotide primers that initiate the reactions. DNA sequencing generally relies on the use of high resolution denaturing polyacrylamide gels which can resolve single stranded DNA ladders over several hundred base pairs.

Maxam-Gilbert sequencing

This method (15) relies on the use of chemical reagents that modify specific bases, followed by the cleavage of the DNA at one or two specific nucleotides. Labeled DNA (usually radioactively labeled at the 3′ or 5′ ends of the strands) is subjected to one of 3 chemical reactions which modify bases in a specific way. Depending on the modification, the chemical piperidine then catalyzes the breakage of DNA at one or two predictable bases. Application of each reaction to adjacent lanes then gives "ladders" which can be deciphered to reveal the DNA sequence. Maxam-Gilbert sequencing, because it uses toxic chemicals, is not the method of choice for large scale sequencing, but it is still used for DNA footprinting where contact sites on DNA are identified.

Dideoxy or chain-termination sequencing (also known as Sanger sequencing)

This is an enzymatic method (16) that relies on the fact that the incorporation of dideoxynucleotides (ddNTPs) rather than deoxynucleotides (dNTPs) results in the termination of elongation of DNA catalyzed by DNA polymerase. DNA polymerases works by elongation of a DNA strand complementary to a template DNA, and requires a hydroxyl (OH) group at the 3′ position for DNA polymerase to add the complementary nucleotides. Since dideoxynucleotides lack a OH group present in deoxynucleotides, the incorporation of a ddNTP terminates elongation.

In dideoxy sequencing, denatured dsDNA or ssDNA is copied (sequenced) using a DNA polymerase. To copy DNA, a DNA polymerase needs a primer and a supply of the 4 bases (dNTPs). A primer is a short oligonucleotide sequence of DNA complementary to one strand that "primes' the process (for dideoxy sequencing, vectors that have so-called "universal priming sites" are generally used). To make the sequence readable, 4 different reactions are used. In each of the 4 different reactions a ddNTP (ddATP, ddCTP, etc.) is added in limiting concentrations. Included in each reaction is a radioactive nucleotide (usually α-^{32}P-dATP is used). The DNA polymerase initiates chain elongation in a 5′ → 3′ direction, starting at 3′ end of the oligonucleotide primer that has been annealed to the DNA template. The DNA polymerase adds deoxynucleotides, which are selected by base-pair matching, to the elongating DNA chain. DNA polymerases can incorporate both dNTPs and ddNTPs as substrates. As a result, chain elongation is terminated whenever a ddNTP is incorporated since they have no 3′ hydroxyl groups. After incubation, the individual reactions containing one of the 4 ddNTPs are run on separate lanes of an acrylamide DNA sequencing gel and then exposed to film. The banding pattern reveals the sequence of the DNA. Figure 2 shows an example of a dideoxy sequencing reaction, with part of the corresponding sequences of two independent clones of a given stretch of DNA. Notice that one of the sequenced clones has a C → G substitution, otherwise known as a mutation.

Figure 2. DNA Sequencing

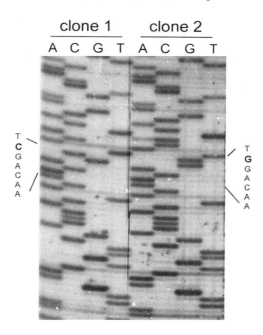

Automated DNA sequencing

Automated sequencing uses the dideoxy sequencing method, but instead of using a radioactive label fluorescent ddNTPs are used, each labeled with a different fluorophore. Once the reactions are completed, they are resolved on a PAGE gel. Because the laser in the automated reader can distinguish the 4 different fluorescent labels, the sequencing can be accomplished by running all 4 reactions in a single lane. Automated sequencing is not only more efficient (more reactions can be loaded on each gel), but generally provides more sequence information per reaction, generating 600–1000 bp or more of readable sequence versus the 300–400 possible with manual sequencing methods.

D. Detection and quantitation of RNA

A number of methods have been developed to identify RNA species and quantify a specific RNA transcript, specifically messenger RNA (mRNA) within total cellular RNA, or total RNA isolated from tissues. mRNA is the "+" or "sense" strand of RNA that is transcribed and processed from DNA encoding a gene that is subsequently translated into protein. The following represent the more commonly employed methods.

Northern blotting

This is a method designed to identify individual RNA that has been fractionated on agarose gels and transferred to a membrane for probing. It is therefore analogous to Southern blotting for DNA. The only major difference is that because RNA can form secondary structures, it must be resolved on gels under denaturing conditions. Common denaturants include formaldehyde and glyoxal.

Northern blotting got its name from its developers, Alwine and Stark (17), who called it "Northern" blotting as a joke (after "Southern" blotting), but the name has stuck, and other blotting methods have since used compass directions as descriptions as well. As for Southern blotting, the probes used are generally DNA probes (cDNA probes, or double stranded genomic DNA fragments that are denatured before use). Northern blotting is commonly used to identify a mRNA transcript in either total cellular RNA or in enriched mRNA. mRNA can be purified using oligo dT cellulose and then fractionated on agarose gels in order to detect rarer transcripts, since most cellular RNA is ribosomal and transfer RNA (tRNA). Northern blots can provide quantitative measures of steady state RNA levels, especially comparative measurements of the relative abundance of RNA in different cell types. However, Northern blotting is not as quantitative as ribonuclease protection assays.

Ribonuclease (RNase) protection assay (RPA)

RPA is used to quantitate steady state levels of RNA, to identify the 5′ or 3′ ends of mRNA, and to characterize the splice junctions of the primary RNA transcripts that are processed into mRNA. The probes used for RPA are RNA probes that are generated by RNA polymerase from bacteriophage promoters, including SP6 (from *Salmonella typhimurium*) and T3 or T7 (from *E. coli*). The DNA to be used for the probe is cloned into a vector downstream of a bacteriophage promoter, and the RNA polymerase is used to produce an RNA probe (usually containing radioactive precursors) complementary to mRNA. Once the RNA probe is hybridized to RNA, RNase is used to remove the free probe and any single stranded segments of hybridizing RNA. The probe will be digested at any point where the probe and RNA do not hybridize. This can be the 5′ end of the RNA, or regions marking exon-intron boundaries. The remaining RNA which was "protected" by annealing to the RNA of interest is then fractionated on a sequencing gel, and the exact size and abundance of the probe remaining can therefore be determined. The size of the protected fragment reveals the start site or domain boundary, while the abundance of the protected fragment reveals the abundance of the RNA transcript.

S1 analysis

S1 analysis is a method used to map exon-intron boundaries and determine the 5′ ends of RNA. S1 analysis usually relies on the use of a single stranded DNA probe that has been labeled on its 5′ end by a kinase. The probe is added to RNA, and the non-hybridizing portion of the probe is digested by S1 nuclease, fractionated by PAGE and analyzed by means similar to RNase protection.

Primer extension

This method is designed to quantitate the levels of a given RNA in a cell as well as to map the 5′ end of the RNA. Primer extension is used to confirm RPA and S1 mapping of the 5′ ends of RNA. Primer extension uses reverse transcriptase (RT; see below) and a primer (a short single stranded DNA) complementary to a sequence in the RNA. After hybridization, the reverse transcriptase (together with dNTP precursors) is used to synthesize ("extend") a cDNA copy of the RNA. Because RT is a polymerase, it synthesizes the cDNA copy in the 5′ → 3′ direction, which is directed toward the 5end of the RNA. Consequently, when the RNA template terminates, extension will end. The length of the cDNA synthesized identifies the length from the primer to the 5′ end of the RNA, and the amount of product synthesized is a direct reflection of the abundance of the RNA.

Other methods to quantitate RNA use modifications of the polymerase chain reaction, and are described in Chapter 3.

Reverse transcriptase (RNA-dependent DNA polymerase)

Reverse transcriptase (RT) is an enzyme isolated from retroviruses (Human Immunodeficiency Virus, or HIV, is one example of a retrovirus). Retroviruses contain a RNA genome, but their life cycle is dependent on the production of a DNA intermediary that integrates into the DNA of the host genome. RT is responsible for transcribing the RNA genome into the first strand of this DNA. A double stranded copy is then synthesized and the proviral DNA is integrated into the host cell genome.

The isolation and characterization of reverse transcriptase was a major breakthrough in our understanding of the life cycle of retroviruses. Its discovery was all the more remarkable since the prevailing wisdom of the time was that DNA was transcribed into RNA, and that the reverse could not (and did not) occur. The identification of RT (18) won the Nobel Prize for its discoverer, David Baltimore, in 1975, which he shared with Renato Dulbecco and Howard Temin for their work on retroviruses and the discovery of tumor viruses.

RT has become an essential tool in biomedical research. In addition to its use in primer extension, RT is used in modified polymerase chain reaction (RT-PCR) studies for quantitative analysis of RNA, for the construction of cDNA libraries, and for differential gene expression studies, to name but a few of its many uses. While the RT used originally was derived from the avian myeloblastosis virus (AMV), a tumor-inducing retrovirus of chickens, most RT used today is genetically modified (one of the many uses of recombinant DNA), removing endogenous RNase activity and enhancing its polymerase activity. These engineered enzymes not only yield more cDNA product, but the cDNAs generated usually are significantly longer and therefore more likely to represent the entire mRNA than the cDNAs generated using native RT.

Like DNA polymerases, RT requires a primer. Oligo dT is frequently used because it hybridizes to the polyA tail characteristic of mRNA. Alternatively, random hexamers (6 bp long random sequences) are used, especially when there is a need to increase the representation of the 5' ends of mRNAs, such as in the production of representative cDNA libraries. No matter how good the RT, many mRNAs cannot be synthesized into intact cDNAs representing the entire mRNA from the 3' end to the 5' end because they are too large.

Chapter 3

RECOMBINANT DNA TECHNIQUES: CLONING AND MANIPULATION OF DNA

A. Introduction

Recombinant DNA refers to DNA that has been experimentally manipulated in a laboratory by adding or deleting genes. Recombinant DNA is usually incorporated into vectors that can be introduced into bacteria, so that the bacteria now contains the gene(s) of interest, genes that they would not normally express. The advent of recombinant DNA technology is one of the most significant developments of 20th century biomedical science. The ability to clone genes led to the establishment of the Biotechnology Industry, which uses cloned genes for enzyme and hormone replacement therapies. For example, before the advent of the biotechnology industry, insulin was purified from natural sources, limiting its availability. Now, it can be produced in essentially limitless quantities and at significantly reduced cost. Recombinant DNA techniques are used to establish new therapies for treating diseases, such as immunodeficiency diseases and metabolic disorders, and are also being used for vaccine development. Recombinant DNA techniques have also significantly enhanced our ability to analyze protein structure and function, determine how genes turn on and off, and understand tissue specific gene expression. The ability to clone DNA allows us to sequence DNA, predict protein structure and experimentally prove function through protein expression and mutagenesis studies. The recombinant DNA revolution has clearly had widespread application in both basic research, and in medical applications.

The first successfully cloned recombinant DNA was by Goff and Berg, who reported the successful construction of hybrid viruses in 1976 (19). In fact, results of the study were known earlier, but their publication was delayed and a moratorium was placed on recombinant DNA technology until a study of its safety could be completed. As a result, most vectors are designed so that they cannot live outside of laboratory conditions. Paul Berg shared the Nobel Prize with Gilbert and Sanger in 1980 for this technological advance.

B.   Plasmid and viral vectors

A vector is a commonly used term for a plasmid or virus that can be used for cloning, expressing and/or transferring DNA from one organism to another. The introduction of DNA sequences from an organism (either prokaryotic or eukaryotic) into a vector is a basic part of recombinant DNA technology. Cloning vectors, whether they are plasmid or viral vectors, contain restriction sites that permit the ligation of foreign DNA into the vector without disrupting sequences necessary for the replication and function of the vector. The type of vector to be used depends on the size and complexity of the DNA to be cloned. For example, cloning genomic DNA requires vectors that can incorporate large pieces of DNA that can only be accommodated by some specialized vectors.

While the recombinant DNA revolution started with the first manipulated cloned DNA in the early 1970's, its genesis really began much earlier. Recombinant DNA technology would not have been possible without previous studies of bacteria and the investigations into the structure and regulation of plasmids and viruses that grow in bacteria, known as bacteriophages. An understanding of the biology of these DNAs and their replication cycles was essential for producing cloned recombinant DNA.

Plasmid

A plasmid is a self-replicating extrachromosomal piece of DNA, which is usually double stranded and circular in nature. Plasmids are naturally found in bacteria where they frequently carry antibiotic resistance markers used by the host bacterium for survival. The accumulation of plasmids accounts for much of the antibiotic resistance evident in new strains of bacteria that are plaguing our hospitals. Plasmids rely on proteins produced by the host bacteria for their replication.

All plasmids used for recombinant DNA work have certain features in common. First, they must be able to replicate, and to do this they contain a replication origin where DNA synthesis begins. Second they must have a selectable marker, so that only the bacteria that contain the plasmid will grow in culture. In general, these are antibiotic resistance genes. Third, they must have a site into which the DNA of interest can be inserted, without affecting the replication or selection of the plasmid. This cloning site contains one or more restriction endonuclease cleavage sites that are not contained elsewhere in the plasmid.

Most commonly used vectors now have a number of unique restriction sites for this purpose in a region called the polylinker or multiple cloning site (MCS). The regions immediately adjacent to the MCS often contain specialized sequences that are used for a variety of purposes, such as providing primer sites for sequencing the inserts (the cloned, inserted DNA), polymerase sites for synthesizing RNA probes from the cloned DNA. These flanking sequences can also contain other modifications that enable the cloned DNA to be expressed in eukaryotic cells, or aid in the analysis of promoter or enhancer activity of the cloned DNA. They may also include additional sequences that permit the construction of fusion proteins (see below). Plasmids used for molecular biology are generally identified with a small "p" at the beginning of their name. Common plasmids include the pBR vectors (pBR322, pBR328, etc.), pUC vectors (pUC18 and pUC19, for example). Vectors within a series can differ in the complexity or orientation of the polylinker, or contain different or additional antibiotic resistance genes. Figure 3 shows an agarose gel

Figure 3. Agarose gel electrophoresis of a restriction digest of a plasmid

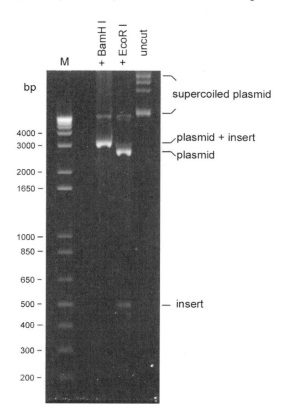

of an uncut plasmid (which reveals the supercoiled plasmid species) or the plasmid digested with a restriction enzyme, BamHI, that "linearizes" the plasmid (cuts one time only) or a restriction enzyme, EcoRI, which is the site into which the insert was cloned. Therefore, after cloning of the insert into the plasmid, there are two EcoRI sites, one on either side of the insert, and the insert "drops out" of the plasmid after digestion, as shown on the gel. M identifies the marker lane, which is a ladder of DNA fragments of know sizes. The marker can be used to calculate the size of the insert.

Transformation

Once a recombinant plasmid is generated, you might be asking how you get it back into the bacterium for its replication. Transformation is the process by which bacterial or plasmid DNA is taken up by a bacterium. Luckily, some bacteria are naturally competent, that is they have evolved ways to take up foreign DNA, such as plasmids. Haemophilus influenzae and Bacillus subtilis are bacterial strains that have evolved natural mechanisms to take up DNA. Bacteria can also be infected by bacteriophages. These processes serve to increase their genetic complexity and improve their survival (as mentioned earlier, plasmids often carry antibiotic resistance genes), and to exchange pieces of their own DNA with the introduced DNA (genetic recombination).

But what about bacteria that are not naturally competent? These strains can be rendered competent experimentally. One bacterial strain that is commonly used in the lab for recombinant DNA work is *Escherichia coli* (*E. coli*). *E. coli* is a rod shaped gram negative bacterium with a circular chromosome that is approximately 3 million base pairs in size. *E. coli* bacteria can be rendered competent by treatment with salts (for example, calcium chloride) or by using a technique called electroporation. Electroporation involves the use of a rapid electric pulse to introduce DNA into a cell. This is thought to function by generating pores in the membrane of the bacterium, which are then repaired. Electroporation can be used for the introduction of DNA into eukaryotic cells as well.

Bacteriophage

A bacteriophage is a virus that infects bacteria. Bacteriophages contain sequences that direct the incorporation of their DNA into phage particles, which can then bind to and infect the bacterium. Bacteriophages are useful as vectors since they generally can accommodate much larger fragments of DNA than plasmids, and can still be successfully "packaged" into an infectious particle. Two types of bacteriophages are commonly employed for recombinant DNA technology, bacteriophage lambda (λ) and its derivatives, and M13. M13 produces, in addition to dsDNA, a single stranded DNA which facilitates DNA sequencing. The introduction of DNA into a bacterium by infection with a bacteriophage is called transduction. The bacteriophages replicate within the bacteria, eventually leading to their destruction (also called lysis), releasing the phage particles, which can then infect adjacent bacteria. When bacteriophages are used to infect a lawn of bacteria grown on an agar plate, they produce viral plaques, which are clear circular regions on the bacterial lawn that result from the lysis of a number of adjacent bacterial by the viral progeny of a single initial infectious virus.

Bacteriophage λ vectors

Bacteriophage λ vectors are useful for the production of **cDNA** libraries and genomic libraries (see below). Bacteriophages are used for the construction of libraries because DNA can be cloned with high efficiency. In addition, these viruses can accommodate large DNA inserts which are much larger than can be cloned into most plasmid vectors. These inserts are packaged into the phage heads. Examples of commonly used bacteriophage λ vectors include λgt10 and λgt11 and the EMBL vectors. λgt10 and λgt11 are used for the high efficiency cloning of cDNA libraries (20). λgt10 is used strictly for the cloning of cDNA libraries, which are screened by hybridization of viral plaques. λgt11 differs from λgt10 in that the cloned DNA is expressed as a stable bacterial fusion protein with β-galactosidase. λgt11 are screened using antibodies specific for a protein of interest. This was at one time the most efficient method of isolating cDNA encoding a particular protein, but other vectors are now available. The cDNA can then be used to identify and characterize the corresponding gene, as well as provide sequence information on the nature of the protein itself.

λEMBL vectors were designed for the cloning and manipulation of genomic DNA (21).

M13 phage vectors

M13 is a family of vectors derived from the bacteriophage M13. These contain a circular, single stranded DNA genome. Once *E. coli* are infected by M13, the phage produces a double-stranded DNA replicative form (RF), which multiplies while continuously producing single stranded phage that are released into the growth media. Because they produce large amounts of single stranded phage which are also easy to isolate, M13 vectors (such as M13mp18) are used for DNA sequencing. However, because they are single stranded, matched pairs of the M13 that produce either a + or − strand of the DNA (*e.g.*, M13mp18 and M13mp19) must be used in order to sequence DNA from both directions. Sequencing from both directions is essential for accurate sequence determination.

M13 phage do not contain a selectable antibiotic resistance marker. However, M13 phage do contain a *lacZ* gene which contains the cloning site. This makes it possible to distinguish bacteriophage that contain DNA inserts from those that do not in the cloning process. The *lacZ* gene, which is a component of the *lac* operon, encodes for the β-galactosidase (β-gal) enzyme. A substrate that can be used for β-gal is X-gal, which turns blue when cleaved by β-gal. As a result, phage in which the *lacZ* gene has been disrupted by an insert will not make the enzyme, and therefore any viral plaques produced will be clear rather than blue. Screening methods using this technique are frequently referred to as "blue-white" screening.

The *lac* operon holds a special place in the study of gene regulation as it was the first genetic system that was understood in prokaryotic cells, specifically *E. coli*. An operon is a set of contiguous genes that are responsible for the synthesis of a particular gene product, often an enzyme and is typical of prokaryotic cells. The operon contains both structural genes and regulatory genes that function both to activate and repress expression. The bacterium *E. coli* lives in lactose-rich environments such as the human gut, and like other cells requires glucose to survive. *E. coli* can convert lactose to glucose using the enzyme β-gal. The lac operon consists of four genes, including *lacZ*, and can turn itself on an off as required, a process known as genetic self-regulation. The *lac* operon was discovered and its function elucidated in the 1960s by Francois Jacob and Jacques Monod, who were awarded the Nobel Prize in Medicine in 1965 for their important contributions to understanding prokaryotic gene regulation.

Phage display

Bacteriophages can also be used to display antibody variable regions, or other proteins or peptides, on their surface, a process known as phage display. This is described in more detail in Chapter 4.

Specialized vectors

In addition to plasmids and phage vectors, there are other vectors that have been developed for specialized use in DNA cloning. Commonly used specialized vectors are described below.

Phagemids

Phagemids are plasmids that contain two different origins of replication. They not only contain their own origin for propagation as a plasmid, but contain a phage origin of replication as well. When a bacterium that contains the plasmid is infected with a "helper phage", the phage origin on the phagemid becomes active. Single stranded DNA is produced from the plasmid DNA and secreted into the bacterial broth. Vector pairs that have the phage origin in opposite direction are available, and as a result single stranded DNA representing both (+ and −) strands of the DNA can be generated.

Examples of phagemids include "Bluescript" vectors (pBluescriptI, pBluescriptII, *etc*.), which are derived from the pUC19 plasmid.

Cosmids

Standard plasmid vectors cannot replicate if large pieces of foreign DNA have been cloned into them, and consequently the use of plasmids is limited to the cloning of DNA inserts that are only a few thousand base pairs. Cosmids were designed to overcome this limitation, so that larger pieces of DNA can be cloned. This is particularly useful in the cloning of intact genes with their corresponding regulatory regions, for example. Cosmids are plasmids that contain a sequence from the lambda phage (known as the cos site) which facilitates the cloning of larger DNA fragments, between 30 and 40 kb in size. Cosmids do, however, have their problems, chief among them the loss of random portions of the inserted DNA.

Artificial chromosomes

In order to be able to clone even larger stretches of DNA, up to 5000 kb (5 million base pairs), vectors have been designed that can accommodate these large DNA pieces. The large size of these cloned fragments allows them to retain many of the structural characteristics of native genomic DNA, including chromatin structure. These cloned fragments of DNA in these vectors are therefore called artificial chromosomes. Two types of artificial chromosomes have been developed, yeast artificial chromosomes (YAC), and bacterial artificial chromosomes (BAC).

A YAC is a plasmid that has been adapted to replicate in yeast. Yeast plasmids are selected using genes that complement mutations in a biosynthetic pathway of yeast, rather than using an antibiotic resistance marker typical of bacterial vectors. Any yeast containing the plasmid will be restored to be able to grow in media that requires the biosynthetic pathway. A BAC plasmid is similar to a YAC vector but is one that can be manipulated in bacteria.

Artificial chromosomes were initially conceived of and developed for use in cloning large fragments of DNA to be used in genome sequencing projects, such as the human genome project. They have now been adapted for a variety of uses, including the identification of segments of chromosomes that encode genes which contribute to human diseases. Artificial chromosomes are also used as a tool to isolate closely linked genes and study their regulation and function in a near normal setting.

Sequencing vectors

These are vectors that are designed to facilitate DNA sequencing. Sequencing vectors contain commonly used primer sites that flank the MCS (SP6 and T7 sequences are common primer sites). In this way, DNA can be sequenced without knowing anything about the sequence of the insert DNA. Many sequencing vectors give rise to single stranded DNA, which is easier to sequence using dideoxy sequencing since it does not have to be denatured before adding the polymerase. DNA sequencing was often carried out using the bacteriophage M13 described earlier. However, phagemids have largely replaced M13 as the vectors of choice for sequencing when single stranded templates are desired. Automated sequencing, however, can easily accommodate double stranded vectors.

Reporter plasmids

These are used to determine if a particular DNA sequence contains transcriptional control regions, including promoter and/or enhancer elements. Reporter plasmids contain a cloning site for the DNA of interest upstream of a reporter gene, a gene whose product can be easily identified. The reporter gene is expressed when the cloned upstream DNA is engaged by transcription factors present in the transfected cell. Expression of the reporter gene implies that transcriptional control regions that are present in the cloned piece of DNA. Early constructs used chloramphenicol acetyltransferase (CAT) as a reporter gene since its enzymatic activity was easy to monitor. In addition, enzymes whose activity can be rapidly detected by spectroscopic methods are frequently used in reporter assays. Popular reporter genes include luciferase (luc; an enzyme isolated from the firefly), or β-gal. The products of these enzymes can be detected spectroscopically, using bioluminescent or chemiluminescent methods, most of which are now automated. Most reporter constructs now contain a gene encoding a "visible" readout, such as green fluorescent protein (GFP). GFP is a protein from the Pacific jellyfish, Aequoria victoria, which fluoresces spontaneously without added substrate. There are a number of variants of GFP that have been genetically engineered to fluoresce at different wavelengths, including yellow fluorescent protein (YFP) and cyan fluorescent protein (CFP).

Expression vectors

Plasmids can be used to express recombinant proteins from both prokaryotic and eukaryotic cells. These "expression vectors" are designed to allow the expression of recombinant DNA sequences in an appropriate host cell. Expression cloning can be used to express a protein at high levels, analyze its function, and identify other proteins with which it interacts, or to investigate its subcellular localization. Expression vectors are similar to conventional plasmids, except the MCS is downstream of an inducible promoter.

Expression vectors are often designed so that the expressed gene is cloned in-frame with a "tag", at either the 5′ or 3′ end. The tag is a sequence that is added to the protein of interest that facilitates both purification and detection. The tag can be detected with an antibody or other specific reagent which then facilitates purification of the fusion protein (a protein that contains two different types of sequences) using affinity chromatography. Some vectors are constructed with an enzyme cleavage site between the expressed protein and the tag, enabling removal of the tag after purification of the fusion protein. Common tags include the FLAG tag, which is an 8 amino acid sequence for which specific antibodies are available; the His tag, which is a sequence encoding 6 consecutive histidine residues that binds nickel with high affinity; and the GST (glutathione-S-transferase) tag, which binds glutathione with high specificity. Each of these types of fusion proteins can be isolated using affinity columns containing the corresponding antibody or ligand, making expression cloning and purification possible even without having an antibody for the protein being cloned.

Eukaryotic expression vectors

These are plasmids that have been adapted for the expression of recombinant proteins in eukaryotic cells. These vectors require the inclusion of a promoter that is activated in the cell in which the gene is to be expressed. Frequently, a promoter that is responsive to ubiquitously expressed transcription factors is included in these vectors, so that they can be used for expression studies in virtually all eukaryotic cells. Common promoters include the beta actin promoter and the cytomegalovirus (CMV) promoter. In addition to a promoter, these vectors may contain enhancer sequences. Eukaryotic expression of a gene requires the presence of an ATG codon (encoding the amino acid methionine) placed in an efficient context for optimal expression of the cloned gene (a Kozak sequence), and a polyadenylation signal sequence downstream of the gene to be expressed. While these can be provided by the cloned gene, most expression vectors contain these sequences.

Transient or stable expression of eukaryotic expression vectors

Eukaryotic expression plasmids can be introduced into cells so that they are expressed in a transient or stable fashion. For transient expression studies, the plasmid is introduced into the cell in its circular form by transfection. A number of transfection methods have been developed, including electroporation of the DNA, adding DNA in the presence of salts (such as calcium chloride) or together with weak base carriers (such as DEAE dextran), or by first incorporating the DNA into lipid vesicles, to name but a few. The plasmid need not replicate, and the eukaryotic gene is expressed for a limited period of time (usually 1 to 3 days). In transient expression studies, only a small fraction of the cells take up and express the transfected DNA.

For stable expression of a DNA in eukaryotic cells, the plasmid is linearized prior to transfection so that it can be incorporated into the host genome. In addition, these vectors contain a selectable marker. A selectable marker is a gene that produces a product that protects cells that have taken up the DNA from an antibiotic that would normally kill the cells. In this way, the cells that have incorporated the transfected DNA can be selected from the bulk of the cells, since the non-transfected cells will die in the presence of the antibiotic. The most frequently used selectable markers are genes encoding the neomycin resistance gene (neo) and the hygromycin resistance gene.

A commonly used eukaryotic expression vector is the pcDNA3 vector used for expressing genes from cDNA. However, many commercial companies have generated expression cloning vectors that contain sequence tags (such as the HIS, FLAG, or GST tags mentioned earlier) or other features to facilitate cloning, detection, or purification of the expressed protein.

Viral vectors

In addition to plasmids, viral vectors can be used to introduce genes into eukaryotic cells. These vectors are often used to increase the frequency of cells expressing the transduced gene (in transient transfection studies) or to introduce the gene into cells that are otherwise refractory to transfection. The three most common forms of viruses that are used are *adenovirus, vaccinia virus, and retroviruses, including lentiviruses. These viral vectors are usually rendered "defective", so that infectious particles are not made in the transduced cells. To render them infectious* for use, these viral vectors must be "packaged" in packaging cell lines in order to make infectious particles.

Baculovirus expression systems

A major drawback of expressing eukaryotic proteins in bacteria is the lack of post-translational processing of the proteins that otherwise occurs in eukaryotic cells. In addition, certain proteins do not fold properly when expressed in prokaryotic (bacterial) cells. To help circumvent these problems, the baculovirus expression system was developed. Baculoviruses are large double stranded DNA viruses that infect insect cells and can express many gene products at high levels. When mammalian genes are expressed using this system, they are usually processed normally and the expressed proteins often form higher level polymers in the same way they are found in mammalian cells, even though the insect cells are grown at 25°–27°C rather than 37°C used for growing mammalian cell lines.

The most common baculovirus used for expressing proteins is *Autographa californica* nuclear polyhedrosis virus, a virus than infects 2 members of the moth family. The insect cell lines commonly used are the SF-9 or SF-21 cell lines, both ovarian cells derived from *Spodoptera frugiperda* (the fall army worm), and High-Five cells from *Trichoplusia ni*, (the cabbage looper). As you might imagine, these cell lines were not developed in medical research settings but borrowed from agricultural research laboratories studying insects!

C.   Libraries

A library is a general term to identify the cloned DNA from an organism, a tissue, or a cell. Two types of libraries are commonly generated, genomic libraries and cDNA libraries. Libraries can be cloned into either plasmids or viruses. Bacteriophages are most commonly used because of their higher cloning efficiency and the ability to package larger-sized DNA inserts into the bacteriophage heads than can be accommodated by plasmids.

Libraries are screened by colony or plaque hybridization or using antibodies as described earlier.

Genomic library

A genomic library is a DNA library containing an organism's genomic DNA. These are commonly used to facilitate the isolation of a gene with its flanking sequences. Genomic libraries are used to isolate and help characterize the intron-exon structure of a gene, and to characterize regulatory domains, including promoter and enhancer elements.

cDNA library

A cDNA library is a library in which the cloned DNA has been synthesized from mRNA expressed by a particular cell, tissue, or organism. The ideal cDNA library contains representatives of all expressed mRNAs in cDNA form at a frequency that is commensurate with the abundance of the expressed mRNA, but such representative cDNA libraries are difficult to achieve. cDNA libraries are frequently used to identify and isolate expressed genes, and to analyze differences in the expression patterns of genes (both known and unknown) in different cell types, in cells at different stages of differentiation, or in different tissues. cDNA libraries can be generated and screened using standard cloning vectors such as λgt0 or they can be screened by expression of a protein using vectors such as λgt11.

In silico cloning

In silico cloning uses computer-based ("in silico") search methods to identify genes. The advantage of *in silico* cloning is that the need for some of the benchwork normally required to clone a gene of interest is bypassed by obtaining as much sequence information as possible from on-line "libraries".

The most useful on-line libraries have been those in the Expressed Sequence Tags (EST) database. The EST database is considered by many to have represented a turning point in genome research. It was first proposed in 1991 as a means to enhance the discovery of new genes and map them in the genome (26). Laboratories from around the world would sample sequence cDNA clones from a variety of libraries and deposit these partial sequences into a central database. This database is part of GenBank (http://www.ncbi.nlm.nih.gov/dbEST/index.html), which is part of the National Center for Biotechnology Information supported by the National Library of Medicine and the National Institutes of Health. Over the years, the database has accumulated millions of partially overlapping and redundant sequences from a variety of organisms. For example there are currently over 5.5 million EST sequences from humans,

4.2 million from the mouse, and tens to hundreds of thousands of sequences from a variety of other organisms. When an investigator identifies a partial sequence from a gene of interest, s/he can screen that sequence against the EST database and obtain additional sequence information for the same or related genes in a single organism, or in different organisms. The EST database has been an invaluable tool to identify the coding sequences in genes that span large amounts of genomic DNA, discover new members of gene families, and identify related genes across species.

D.   Site Directed Mutagenesis

Introduction

Specific mutations in the DNA sequence of genes can result in the loss of function of the encoded protein. The classical way of defining gene function is to select for phenotypic changes, and then correlate these with specific mutations. However, this is cumbersome and slow, since the rate of mutation in genes is low (1 in 10^6 base pairs per generation) and many changes do not result in perceptible phenotypic changes in the corresponding protein. A more rapid and productive method of introducing changes in genes is to experimentally mutate the gene, and then test for changes in function that result from these mutations. This method, called site directed mutagenesis, was the brainchild of Michael Smith, who shared the Nobel Prize with K. Mullis in 1993 for this landmark idea (22). Using site directed mutagenesis, one or more nucleotides can be altered in a gene, resulting in changes in the corresponding amino acid sequence of the encoded protein. Today, site directed mutagenesis is used routinely to identify and characterize important regulatory elements of genes and to identify individual domains and specific amino acids within protein domains that are responsible for their function. The rapid advancement in our understanding of how enzymes function, the identification of the templates recognized by enzymes, an understanding of how proteins interact with each other or with their cognate DNA sequences (in the case of transcription factors), the determination of motifs in proteins that are crucial for protein folding and their three-dimensional structures, and the "quality control" mechanisms within a cell that govern protein folding and retention in the secretory pathway. All of these advances can be traced to a large extent to the invention and use of site directed mutagenesis.

Site directed mutagenesis is one of the most powerful methods available for the analysis of protein structure:function relationships using recombinant DNA technology. It also has advanced possibilities of

constructing proteins with improved stability or with totally new properties. Antibodies with improved specificity and affinity can be generated
for therapeutic purposes using site directed mutatagenesis (see Chapter 4). Several methods have been developed for mutating cloned genes.
The most commonly used are briefly described below.

Oligonucleotide-directed mutagenesis

This method allows for the alteration of a DNA sequence in a specific
way, and was invented by M. Smith. An oligonucleotide with a mutation of
interest is hybridized to the corresponding template sequence in plasmid
or viral DNA, and extended using DNA polymerase. If a circular DNA
template, such as a plasmid, or single stranded phage template such
as M13 is used, the second strand DNA will extend to the primer and
DNA ligase can be used to ligate the DNA product, producing a double
stranded product. The DNA is then used to transform competent *E. coli*
bacteria. The mismatch is then repaired in bacterial cells, which fixes
the mutation for selection using standard recombinant DNA techniques.
The function of the mutant gene can then be tested by expressing it
in the appropriate cells or in an organism.

A variation of this method uses "degenerate" oligonucleotides cov-
ering the region of interest (these are synthesized by adding small
amounts of incorrect nucleotide precursors during synthesis of the
oligonucleotide). The mixture of oligonucleotides is annealed to the template, double stranded DNA is synthesized, and individual clones are
isolated and characterized.

PCR-directed mutagenesis

This is a variation of oligonucleotide-directed mutagenesis, in which
oligonucleotides containing mutations of interest are used as primers
in a polymerase chain reaction (see below for explanation of PCR).
The primers often contain restriction sites (either native to the gene or
introduced for cloning purposes). The resulting DNA is then cloned using
standard methods.

Linker scanning mutagenesis

This is a method for introducing a number of clustered mutations in a
short stretch of DNA. It is primarily used to identify transcriptional regulatory regions of a gene. Generally, linker scanning mutants are generated
that contain individual clusters over a larger region in order to rapidly determine which region(s) are important in regulating a gene's expression.

E.   Polymerase chain reaction (PCR)

Introduction

The polymerase chain reaction is a method used for amplifying DNA sequences *in vitro*. It is elegant in its simplicity, and yet its many uses have revolutionized the life sciences. It has almost unlimited applications in the biomedical sciences, genetics, and biotechnology, and is an important tool in forensics as well. PCR even has applications to anthropology and archaeology. For its invention, Kary Mullis, who conceptualized the process in 1983 on a drive to his mountain cabin in California, shared the Nobel Prize in Chemistry in 1993. At the time, he was trying to help solve the problem of how to develop a diagnostic test for a genetic disease, sickle cell anemia, that resulted from by a single base pair mutation in the hemoglobin gene. The solution, PCR, was published in 1985 (23). The background for the invention of the PCR was recounted by Mullis in **Scientific American** (24).

There are several forms of PCR, all of which incorporate the three basic steps of the PCR reaction (Figure 4). First, the dsDNA is denatured to separate it into two single strands. Second, the "primer" is allowed

Figure 4.   Polymerase chain reaction

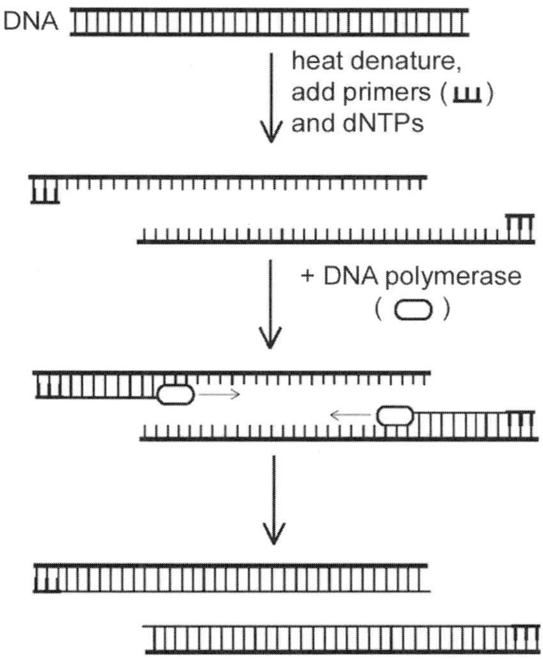

to anneal by lowering the temperature. Third, the reaction is "extended" by a polymerase; the temperature of this reaction is usually between the other two. In its simplest form, PCR starts with two short oligonucleotide primers, each of which is complementary to opposite strands of the DNA. The DNA is heat denatured to separate the strands, and as the temperature is lowered, the primers anneal to the DNA. In the presence of DNA polymerase and each of the 4 dNTPs, copies of each strand are produced. The sample is heated again, the temperature lowered to allow annealing with the PCR primers, and the process is repeated. The amplification process doubles the amount of DNA synthesized from the two primers at each step, each of which takes a couple of minutes. As a result, in an hour or two, 30 rounds of PCR can be carried out, resulting in more than a billion copies of a specific region of DNA from a single DNA template ($2^{30} = 1,073,741,824$, to be exact!). The DNA needs not be abundant or pure. This is why DNA can be typed from a single human hair or drop of blood. Small amounts of DNA have been extracted from mummies, as well as from animals frozen in glaciers tens of thousands of years ago. PCR allows this DNA to be compared to their counterparts of today. And, as you might have guessed, DNA has been extracted from insects preserved in amber and amplified by PCR, a process that formed the basis of Michael Crichton's book, **"Jurassic Park",** and the subsequent movies.

In its original incarnation, new DNA polymerase had to be added at each step of PCR since the temperature used to separate the DNA strands (commonly $94°C$, which is near boiling) also inactivated the enzyme. This problem was solved when a DNA polymerase that was stable at high temperatures was isolated from the bacterium *Thermus aquaticus* (Taq polymerase) which thrives in hot springs. Today, a number of genetically engineered heat stable DNA polymerases are available for use in PCR, and the PCR reaction is carried out in programmable instruments that rapidly heat and cool samples for each round of amplification.

PCR has been adapted to a number of uses in biomedical sciences. In some cases, nested PCR primers are used, particularly when the template DNA is in low abundance. Nested primers are primers in which a first pair of oligonucleotides is used to amplify DNA for a number of rounds, and then a second pair of primers (located within the bounds of the first PCR product) is used for further amplification. This not only allows for the amplification of small amounts of DNA, but sometimes significantly improves specificity.

A small sampling representing the most common variations of PCR are outline below.

Reverse transcription PCR (RT-PCR)

PCR is used to detect DNA sequences but it can be adapted to identify RNA in a sample as well. To this end, reverse transcriptase is added together with a reverse primer and nucleotides to generate a cDNA. The sample, or an aliquot of the sample, is then subjected to standard PCR procedures. This has proved to be a relatively simple and rapid method to determine if a particular gene is expressed in a cell or cell population.

Semiquantitative PCR

PCR is extremely sensitive and can easily amplify a single DNA segment. However, standard PCR is not quantitative. While in theory there should be a relationship between the amount of starting material and the final product, in practice this is not always the case. Semiquantitative PCR was established to overcome this deficiency. The development of semiquantitative and quantitative PCR has been an especially significant advancement in our ability to ascertain the level of expression of a gene in different cells and tissues.

A common method of generating semiquantitative RT-PCR data is to analyze the products after varying numbers of PCR cycles (Figure 5). This allows the investigator to identify the quantitative portion of the amplification cycles. In the example shown, the products are visualized every 3 cycles of PCR beginning at 21 cycles, so that the amount of DNA generated should increase 8-fold between samples. By comparing the amount of product from the same number of cycles from two different types of cells, (and standardizing them with products from genes that are expressed at similar levels in the two cells), an investigator can determine the relative abundance of mRNA for that particular gene in the two cell types. This method is at least as quantitative as Northern blot analysis and RPA, and can be accomplished more quickly and with smaller amounts of starting material.

Figure 5.   Semiquantitative polymerase chain reaction

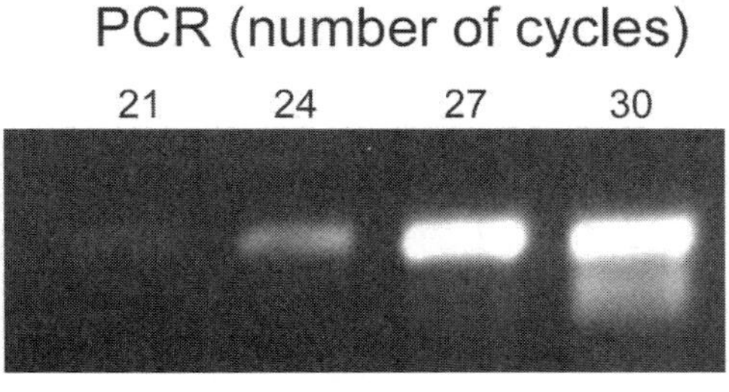

PCR (number of cycles)

Quantitative real-time PCR

The most sensitive and quantitative approach to PCR is through the use of "real-time" PCR. The basis for real-time PCR is to utilize a system that permits the detection of a PCR product as it accumulates in the reaction. Real-time PCR can be used experimentally or clinically, for example to determine the viral load in an HIV-infected individual. The first real-time PCR used the fluorescent properties of ethidium bromide, which binds quantitatively to DNA as it is produced (25). Several fully automated real-time PCR systems have now been developed. These include a thermal cycler, a light source (often a laser) to induce fluorescence, a CCD "charged coupled detector" camera for detection and, of course, computer software to graphically translate the information collected. Although the different technologies vary somewhat, they have in common the ability to sample and detect in real-time a fluorescent product generated during PCR. By comparing this product with the amplification of a housekeeping genes (beta-actin is commonly used), true quantitative comparisons between samples can be accomplished, providing accurate measurements of the initial quantity of mRNA or DNA in different samples. A major advantage of quantitative real-time PCR systems is that the instrumentation provides the readout, and no gel electrophoresis is required to analyze the PCR product.

One type of quantitative PCR uses the TaqMan® probe system. The TaqMan probe system is based on FRET (fluorescence resonance energy transfer) principles, in which the close proximity of two fluorescent dyes that can transfer energy results in fluorescence quenching (see Chapter 5 for more information). In the TaqMan probe system, a specially designed oligonucleotide probe that contains two fluors, the reporter and a quencher, hybridizes to the fragment being extended by PCR. As the PCR product is extended, the 5′ exonuclease activity of the Taq polymerase digests the probe, releasing the reporter from the quencher, resulting in fluorescence. As the product is amplified, the fluorescence increases quantitatively.

A second type of system uses the dye SYBR Green, which is a highly specific dsDNA binding dye that remains associated with the DNA generated during the PCR amplification. Standard primers are used to amplify DNA and the SYBR Green fluorescence is detected and plotted during the amplification process. At the linear portion of the curve (when plotted as $\log_{10}$ fluorescence vs the number of rounds of PCR), a comparison of the number of rounds of PCR required to give a constant amount of fluorescence can give quantitative comparisons between samples. This type of real-time PCR is especially useful for ChIP analysis (see chromatin immunoprecipitation section below).

Ligation-mediated PCR (LM-PCR)

LM-PCR is a method used for analyzing the sequence and characteristics of short stretches of genomic DNA, such as when identifying protein-DNA footprints *in vivo*. In LM-PCR, single stranded breaks in the DNA are created, using Maxam-Gilbert reactions for example. After conversion of a break to a blunt-end duplex, an oligonucleotide primer (which has a linker associated with it) is ligated to the blunt end, and PCR amplification is carried out. The product can then be detected by Southern blotting or by visualization using ethidium bromide staining after another round of PCR is carried out, using an internal (nested) primer.

Methylation-specific PCR (MSP)

This method is used to determine the methylation pattern of cytosine residues in genomic DNA. Cytosine residues are often methylated in regions of DNA that are rich in CpG dinucleotides. Highly methylated genes are often not expressed, and aberrant methylation patterns are often associated with the inappropriate expression (or repression) of genes in malignant cells. MSP is used to determine methylation patterns of regulatory regions, such as promoters and enhancers, which often correlate with transcriptional status of the corresponding gene. MSP relies on the sequence differences between methylated and unmethylated DNA that occurs when the DNA is treated with sodium bisulfite (bisulfite converts non-methylated, but not methylated, cytosines to uracil). PCR is then used to amplify the DNA using primers specific for methylated and unmethylated DNA in the region of interest.

F. Screening for differentially expressed genes (DEGs)

Differential screening

What makes a lymphocyte a lymphocyte, and not a muscle or nerve cell? What makes a B lymphocyte what it is, and not a T lymphocyte? And what changes in gene expression occur as a cell becomes more differentiated? These are questions that can be approached by identifying differentially expressed genes. The identification of mRNA transcripts that are expressed in one tissue but not another, or is expressed at higher abundance, is a first step to understanding what makes cells at different stages of development unique. It has been estimated that no more than 10% to 20% of the genes in the genome may be expressed at any given time in a tissue. Some of the expressed genes will be "house-keeping" genes, expressed in all tissues, and others may be responsible for the development or function of a particular cell type. Together with transcriptional profiling, differential screening is a powerful tool to understand lineage specific gene expression. However, identification of a differentially expressed gene is only the first step. Once identified, the important task is determining what the function(s) of these genes might be the developmental fate or function of the cells. This is no small task!

So how many genes are there? With the completion of the Human Genome Project (and the completion of the sequencing of other mammalian genomes, including mouse and rat), one might have thought that this would be a simple question. However, estimates of the number of genes vary dramatically, from 24,000 to 75,000 genes, depending in part on the algorithms used for the estimates. Most geneticists believe the lower number is accurate and, if true, it means that humans only have about 4,000 more genes than the simple nematode, *Caenorhabditis elegans (C. elegans)* a species that is frequently used as a model system to study the role of genes in cell fate development.

There are a number of methods that have been developed over the years to isolate and identify differentially expressed genes. Many of these methods rely on screening cDNA libraries at some point. Each of them have a number of drawbacks, and each comes with its own set of artifacts. Nevertheless, these have proven to be powerful tools to help scientists understand the role that differential gene expression has in development and differentiation of cells and tissues.

Subtractive hybridization (also known as subtractive cloning)

This was one of the first methods developed to identify differentially expressed genes. This method is based on the ability of complementary DNA (cDNA) to specifically hybridize to messenger RNA (mRNA). In its simplest form, a large molar excess (10 to 100 fold) of mRNA from one cell population (cell A) is hybridized to cDNA from another cell (cell B), and the DNA-RNA hybrids removed. In theory, cDNAs that remain un-hybridized represent transcripts of genes that are expressed in higher abundance in cell type B. These can be used directly to screen a cDNA library, or used as templates for generating double stranded cDNAs and cloned. The resultant library represents differentially expressed genes. Like all subtractive methods, subtractive hybridization is fraught with artifacts, and consequently the differential expression of any cloned gene needs to be confirmed by a second method. A common method is to use the subtracted clone as a probe in Northern blots of mRNA from cells A and B.

Differential display

Differential display is a PCR-based method to amplify differentially expressed genes. mRNA from the two cell types to be compared is first reverse transcribed into cDNA using oligo(dT) based primers, and then these cDNAs are amplified with a set of short, random primers. The bands generated by the primer sets from each cell type are then compared on high resolution gels (denaturing polyacrylamide "sequencing" gels are generally employed). The investigator then compares (literally using the stare and compare method) the band patterns. Unique bands found in one sample but not the other sample using the same sets of primers, or bands represented at significantly different abundances, are considered to be candidates for differentially expressed genes. To identify the mRNA represented by the candidate band, the band can be sequenced and databases searched for the corresponding sequence (the preferred method), or it can be excised from the gel and used to probe cDNA libraries.

Representation difference analysis (RDA)

RDA is a method that combines subtractive hybridization with PCR amplification to enrich for differences in genomes between two closely related species or to enrich for differences in expressed genes between two different tissues or cell types. Genomic DNA or cDNA from the two DNA samples to be compared are digested with a restriction enzyme that is a "frequent cutter", and linkers are added to the DNA. Linkers are short, double-stranded oligonucleotides that contain a restriction site. In theory, PCR amplification using sequences in the linkers allows for the unbiased amplification of the DNA samples, a critical step for subtractive hybridization when comparisons are to be meaningful. Following amplification, the linkers are then removed from both populations of DNA. New linkers are added to one source of amplified DNA (the tester). Small amounts of the tester are added to a large excess of the second DNA (the driver) and melted (which generates denatured single stranded DNA). The DNA is then allowed to hybridize. Only the DNAs present in excess in the tester will rehybridize to itself, resulting in a small subset of DNAs that have linkers on both strands since the excess driver will hybridize with most of the tester DNA. This small subset can then be amplified and cloned for analysis.

Serial analysis of gene expression (SAGE)

SAGE is a method that was designed to provide a relative quantitation and unbiased analysis of the genes expressed in a cell rather than differences between cells. It involves the production of short (14 bp) cDNA fragments upstream the poly(A) tail of the expressed mRNA, a size that has been calculated to be sufficient to identify the gene from which it is expressed. These tags are concatemerized, cloned and amplified in bacteria. These cloned tags can then be sequenced "en masse" to identify the expressed genes in the cell.

DNA microarrays

While other methods for accomplishing differential screening described above are still useful, the advent of DNA microarrays, also known as DNA chips or gene chips, have revolutionized the ability to rapidly identify differences in the expression of genes between different cells and tissues. DNA microarrays are arrays containing a large number of samples of DNA that represent many if not all of the known genes in a given species, tethered to the array matrix in a known order. The DNA samples on the matrix are either cDNAs (in sizes of a few hundred to a few thousand bp) or oligonucleotides 20–80 bp in length representing each of the known genes. The matrix is usually glass, but nylon substrates are also used. Current technology using robotic fabricators allows for the covalent attachment of 30,000 to 60,000 individual oligonucleotides to a single matrix, providing (in theory) one or more representatives of each of the thousands of expressed genes in the human genome. DNA microarrays are available for the human, mouse and rat genomes, and microarrays representing a number of pathogens have also been produced.

The microarrays are probed with cDNAs that have been synthesized from a sample of RNA incorporating a fluorescent nucleotide. The labeled cDNA can then be used to probe the matrix, and the hybridized species are detected by an sophisticated array reader to determine which of the genes on the matrix are expressed in the RNA sample. Since the genes of any species can be represented on one or two microarrays, an investigators can now determine which genes are expressed in any given cell or tissue within the matter of a couple of days!

However, the capabilities and uses of DNA microarrays are even greater! With the help of powerful computer programs (the analysis of microarray data is computationally intensive and generates more data than can be easily interpreted without the aid of computers), information from DNA microarrays can be used to compare the expressed genes in two (or more) different samples. This allows an investigator not to determine which genes are expressed, but to compare the relative abundance of gene expression in the different samples. This has proven critical to following gene expression during development and differentiation of tissues and cells, and has in the last few years been applied to analysis of cancerous tissues. Importantly, these gene profiling studies have allowed investigators to identify gene expression patterns that can distinguish between tumors that were once thought to be identical, and yet responded differently to therapy. These profiles can not only be used to predict how a person with a tumor will respond to therapy, but may ultimately provide new insights into the development of new therapeutics for cancers refractory to treatment.

G. Promoter-protein interactions

Introduction

The human body is made up of over 200 types of cells, each of them distinct. While they all contain the same genetic information, they each developed as a result of the programming of a distinct subset of genes. What makes a muscle a muscle and not a nerve is determined by the pattern of gene expression prior to and during development, as well as by the set of genes that are expressed in the differentiated cell. The control of gene expression is a complex process that not only requires that the promoter and enhancer elements that regulate expression are "accessible" to transcription factors, but that the required transcription factors are present. Determining which *cis* elements in a gene serve as transcriptional control elements (the promoters and enhancers) requires methods that can identify these sequences. Once identified, the identity of the transcription factors that bind the sequences can be identified. The following sections briefly outline some of the most common methods employed.

Reporter assays

Reporter constructs are used to determine if a sequence of DNA can act as a promoter or enhancer in a particular cell. The way that reporter plasmids are constructed has been outlined in an earlier section. These can be transiently transfected into the cell of interest, and promoter activity measured using one of several "readouts" described earlier including the production of luciferase, or β-gal or CAT activity. It is important to remember that even if a particular sequence upstream of a gene shows promoter activity in this type of assay it does not necessarily mean that it is a promoter! Plasmids generally expose "naked" DNA, devoid of histones and nucleosomal structures common to DNA present in chromosomes. Therefore, it is important to determine the "accessibility" of the DNA in the cell using other methods (see below).

Electrophoretic mobility shift assay (EMSA)

An EMSA or **band shift** is used to detect the interactions between DNA binding proteins (including transcription factors) and a DNA sequence recognized by those proteins. This method was developed in 1981 (27) as a rapid and semiquantitative method for identifying protein interactions with specific DNA sequences. EMSA works well with crude nuclear extracts from cells or purified proteins produced by recombinant DNA methods. Extracts or purified proteins are incubated with a radiolabeled (^{32}P) dsDNA probe containing the putative recognition site. The dsDNA can come from cloned DNA from a putative promoter or enhancer sequence, or oligonucleotides containing known protein binding motifs (or mutations of these). The DNA-protein complexes are then separated from the free probe by nondenaturing PAGE, and the gel is exposed to film. While the free probe will migrate rapidly, the bound probe will be "retarded" in the gel and migrate more slowly. Figure 6

Figure 6.   Electrophoretic mobility shift assay

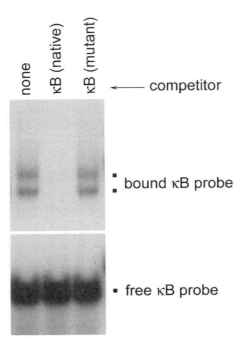

shows an example of an EMSA using a probe that contains a binding site, called $_\kappa$B, which interacts with a family of transcription factors collectively called NF-$_\kappa$B. The two shifted bands represent the binding of two different NF-$_\kappa$B complexes. To prove specificity of binding in EMSA assays, competition experiments are performed. First, the binding of the extracts can be performed in the presence of "cold" competitors (an unlabeled identical probe added in excess), which demonstrates that the shift is not nonspecific. Second, when a mutant probe with an identical sequence except in the DNA binding site is used as a cold competitor, binding is not inhibited.

To identify the DNA binding proteins in nuclear extracts that are bound to the DNA probe, antibodies specific for known transcription factors can be used. Two common methods employing specific antibodies for this purpose are the supershift assay and UV cross-linking and immunoprecipitation.

Supershift assay

This is a variation of the EMSA in which antibodies are used to identify specific proteins associated with DNA probes used in EMSA. After binding of nucleic acids to the radioactive probe, antibodies to specific proteins are added to the complex. If the protein is present, the migration of the complex will be altered. Specifically, the presence of the antibody will further retard the migration of the complex, resulting in a band on the gel that migrates more slowly than the corresponding band without the antibody. As a result, the band appears shifted up, hence the name "supershift". Note, however, that some antibodies cannot be used for this supershift assays since some can disrupt the binding of the protein to the DNA.

Supershift assays are important not only to confirm the identity of the protein interacting with a DNA sequence, but also are useful to identify proteins in complexes that do not necessarily interact with the DNA. While active transcription complexes consist of proteins that interact directly with specific DNA templates, they often contain other proteins that interact with these proteins (via protein-protein interactions). Examples of these include coactivators. Supershift assays provide one way to detect some of these additional proteins, although large complexes are not frequently resolved by either standard EMSA or supershift assays.

UV-crosslinking and immunoprecipitation

In this variation of the EMSA, nuclear extracts are incubated with the dsDNA template, and then the proteins that are bound to the DNA are cross-linked to it. These are then immunoprecipitated with specific antibodies, the cross-link reversed, and the proteins identified on conventional SDS-PAGE gels by western blotting.

DNA footprinting

DNA footprinting is a method for identifying the sites on the DNA that are recognized by DNA-binding proteins. There are a number of different DNA footprinting methods that allow for the detection of DNA binding proteins under a variety of conditions. One of the most common footprinting methods is DNase I footprinting. The DNA from a restriction fragment is labeled at one end with ^{32}P and is subjected to partial hydrolysis by DNase I in the presence and absence of the bound protein. The fragments produced will be different at the site of binding because the bound protein will protect the DNA from cleavage. The protected site is visualized as a gap in the ladder, the footprint, which identifies the region bound by the protein.

Chromatin immunoprecipitation (ChIP)

ChIP is a method used to examine whether a particular protein is bound to a given DNA sequence *in vivo*. Unlike EMSAs, which determine whether a particular transcription factor CAN bind to a DNA sequence, ChIP assays can reliably tell an investigator IF a DNA sequence is occupied by a protein of interest under physiological conditions. In this method, DNA-binding proteins are cross-linked to DNA (using formaldehyde), the chromatin is isolated and sheared into fragments with their accompanying bound proteins. Specific antibodies are then used to immunoprecipitate the bound proteins with their corresponding DNA sequences. The cross-linking is reversed and, to determine if the DNA of interest has been immunoprecipitated, specific PCR primers are used to amplify the DNA.

Biotinylated DNA pulldown assays

This assay was developed to help improve the ability to identify larger protein complexes associated with particular DNA sequences. In this assay, biotinylated DNA (DNA can be biotinylated on the 5′ ends of each DNA strand) is incubated with nuclear extracts. The complex can be removed from other proteins ("pulled down") in the extracts using streptavidin-agarose beads. The proteins can then be dissociated from the complex using SDS-PAGE sample buffer and resolved on these gels.

The presence of specific proteins can then be identified by western blot analysis.

Southwestern blot

A southwestern blot is one method that is sometimes used to identify DNA-binding proteins, and characterize their binding specificity. Nuclear proteins, purified from nuclei isolated from homogenized cells are resolved by SDS-PAGE, transferred to a membrane and probed with oligonucleotide probes. The oligonucleotides that are used can correspond to consensus DNA motifs recognized by defined transcription factors, or their mutant counterparts. This method works for some, but not many, DNA binding proteins because the DNA binding sites often depend on three-dimensional folding patterns that are often disrupted during protein processing.

Yeast two-hybrid screen

The yeast two-hybrid system is a powerful system for identifying interacting transcriptional activators. It was described in detail in Chapter 1.

H.   Silencing gene expression

Introduction

A number of approaches are used to determine the function of a gene. cDNA encoding a gene can be expressed in cells in wild-type and mutant forms, using site-directed mutagenesis. However, it is often desirable to produce a functional knockout of a gene in order to determine the effect that the failure to express a particular gene has cellular function. Knockouts can be accomplished in several different ways. First, a gene can be functionally deleted in embryonic stem cells by homologous recombination, and the deletion introduced into the germline in animals. This is discussed in Chapter 6. Methods have also been developed to functionally inactivate a gene's expression using knockdown or gene silencing approaches. These methods can be used in certain organisms and in some, but not all cell types. These methods are briefly described below.

Antisense RNA

Antisense RNA is a method that attempts to block translation of mRNA by introduction of a corresponding minus strand nucleic acid into the cell. The minus strand nucleic acid can be introduced by transfection of plasmid from which minus strand (and thus "antisense") RNA is synthesized, or by introducing single stranded cDNA oligonucleotides into the cell. The theory is that the antisense RNA or cDNA forms duplexes with the mRNA and consequently inhibits translation. This is thought to be accomplished by preventing the ribosome from gaining access to the mRNA or by increasing the rate of degradation of the duplexed mRNA. In either event, the failure to translate the protein provides an opportunity for an investigator to test for changes in the cell that result from the lack of gene expression. Obviously, this method works only if the endogenous protein in the cell is relatively short-lived!

RNA interference (RNAi)

RNAi is a naturally occurring phenomenon but can also be used as a method of gene silencing. RNAi has been used in a number of intact organism including the nematode *C. elegans*, where this method was first discovered, as well as in fruit flies and plants. RNAi begins with long, double-stranded RNA molecules (usually larger than 200 nt), which are enzymatically cleaved by an RNase called "dicer" in the cell to 22 bp molecules, which are called small interfering RNAs (siRNA). The RNA is assembled into complexes that lead to the unwinding of the siRNA, which hybridizes with mRNA and inhibits its translation, presumably by causing its cleavage and destruction. Molecular details of these processes remain poorly understood.

RNAi does not work effectively in mammalian cells because the introduction of dsRNA into these cells can lead to an antiviral response due to the recognition of the RNA by certain receptors involved in the innate immune response, called Toll-like receptors (TLR). However, the introduction of the shorter siRNA into some, but not all, mammalian cells can lead to gene silencing. In these cells this provides a potent means to study gene function in these cells.

I.   Forensics and DNA technology

Introduction

Most of us are aware of real-life situations where DNA typing has been used to attempt to solve a murder (who can forget "the OJ case"?). The significant use of DNA techniques has even made it into our entertainment culture, as exemplified by the popularity of TV programs like the "CSI: Crime Scene Investigation" series. But what methods are used for identification of DNA samples to match them to a particular individual?

Any two humans differ by about 0.1% of their genome, representing about 3 million of the 3 billion base pairs in the human genome. To compare the DNA of a suspect with DNA obtained at a crime scene, the investigator must use methods that take advantage of these differences to generate a unique DNA profile for comparing samples.

RFLP

One method that can be used is RFLP (restriction fragment length polymorphisms; see Chapter 2) analysis. By comparing 4 or 5 known RFLPs, a forensic scientist can readily exclude or include a suspect with DNA obtained at a crime scene. RFLP requires a significant amount of DNA, more than normally found at a crime scene in "pristine" condition.

PCR

Because RFLP cannot be used reliably, PCR techniques are more commonly employed, since this allows an investigator to amplify and analyze small amounts of DNA. The major problem with PCR is that even minute amounts of material that might have contaminated the sample during its identification or collection can raise doubt about the conclusions of the investigator.

Short tandem repeat (STR)

Short tandem repeat (STR) analysis is a very common method of analyzing specific loci in genomic DNA. STRs commonly are composed of repeats of 2 to 5 nucleotides in a "head to tail" manner (for example, gatagatagata represents 3 gata repeats). STRs can be found on different chromosomes and vary significantly between individuals. The CODIS (COmbined DNA Index System) database, which was established by Congress in 1994 for the use of the FBI and local and state governments to identify sex offenders, uses a core of 13 STRs to distinguish between individuals. The odds that any two individuals are identical at the 13 STRs are about 1 in a billion.

Other markers

Two other sets of markers are useful in identifying the DNA profile of an individual. These include mitrochondrial DNA analysis and Y chromosome analysis. Mitochondrial DNA is often used when nuclear DNA, which is required for RFLP and STR analysis, cannot be extracted with confidence. The mitochondria, bacteria-like organelles within each cell that generate much of the energy required by the cell, are transmitted in a manner distinct from nuclear DNA. Mitochondrial DNA is always maternally transmitted; consequently, DNA from missing person investigations can be compared with a maternal relative for identification. The analysis of genetic markers on the Y chromosome aids in the identification of males since the Y chromosome is transmitted from father to son.

It should be noted that these methods are not just useful for crime scene investigative purposes, but can be used to trace ancestry as well. For example, Y chromosome analysis was used to compare the DNA of descendents of Thomas Jefferson (yes, our third president) and those of his slave Sally Hemings. This analysis provided the first conclusive evidence in support of the theory that the two had at least one child together while President Jefferson was in his second term of office (28).

Chapter 4

ANTIBODY-BASED TECHNIQUES

A.   Introduction

Antibodies are a group of serum glycoproteins of related structure that help protect us against invading pathogens. Antibodies are highly specific for the immunogen, and generally bind with high affinity to antigenic determinants, known as epitopes, on the immunogen. Antibodies that have been produced against an immunogen can be purified from serum using, for example, affinity chromatography. These purified antibodies are generally heterogeneous in that they recognize different epitopes on the immunogen and bind with different affinities. These serum antibodies are referred to as polyclonal antibodies since they have been produced by many different clones of antibody secreting cells. Antibody secreting cells, also referred to as plasma cells, differentiate from B lymphocytes in response to foreign antigens. Antibodies are crucial to the clearance of many pathogens like viruses and bacteria from our bodies. The most remarkable feature of antibodies is their ability to be produced against almost any type of macromolecule, especially proteins and carbohydrates, whether these are naturally occurring or synthesized *de novo* in the laboratory.

Major discoveries on the role of antibodies in adaptive immune responses have been met with a number of Nobel prizes to investigators during the 20th century (see Table 3). However, antibodies have also become one of the most important tools in biomedical research because of their ease of production and characteristic specificity and affinity.

There are a number of different isotypes (also called classes) of antibodies that have distinct biologic activities. In most mammals there are 5 isotypes, IgM, IgG, IgA, IgE, and IgA. The biologic activities of these antibody classes are quite varied. While some pathogens, especially viruses, may be inactivated by antibody binding, most are not destroyed

Table 3.   Selected Nobel Laureates (antibodies and immune function)

Emil Adolf von Behring	discovery of antibodies; use of serum therapy for treatment of infections (anti-toxins)	1901[†]
Ilya Ilyich Mechnikov Paul Ehrlich	discovery of phagocytosis; theories relating to self-non-self discrimination	1908[†]
Jules Bordet	discovery of complement; proof that antibodies can be made against benign foreign antigens	1919[†]
Karl Landsteiner	chemical nature of antigens; discovery of blood groups*	1930[†]
Gerald M. Edelman Rodney R. Porter	discovery of the structure of antibodies	1972[†]
Rosalyn Yalow (Roger Guillemin, Andrew V. Schally)	development of RIA technology to quantitate peptide hormones (discovery of peptide hormones)	1977[†]
Niels K. Jerne Georges J.F. Köhler César Milstein	theories on specificity of the immune system (Jerne); invention of monoclonal antibody technology	1984[†]
Susumu Tonegawa	discovery of the genetic basis of antibody diversity	1987[†]

[†]Nobel Prize in Physiology or Medicine
*Lansteiner suggested that blood groups could be used in forensics and for paternity testing.

unless antibody effector functions are activated. One effector function is the activation of complement, which is activated by some antibody isotypes. Complement is name for a number of serum proteins that can destroy invading pathogens by lysing them. Complement causes lysis by the insertion of proteins into the membrane which form pores, thereby causing the loss of cellular integrity. Complement activation also results in the production of chemoattractants, which are small bioactive cleavage products of the complement cascade whose production elicits the accumulation of specific white blood cells (including macrophages and neutrophils) that engulf and destroy pathogens. Certain antibody classes can cross the placenta to protect the fetus, or cross the epithelial layers to get into secretions to fight pathogens before they enter sterile spaces of the body. The constant region domains of some antibodies are bound by cellular receptors on phagocytic cells after antibody binding to pathogens, which causes the uptake and destruction of the pathogens. Antibodies are also responsible for our allergies, but this same antibody class (IgE) also helps destroy parasites.

Each antibody isotype is an oligomeric glycoprotein composed of two heavy chains and two light chains (two classes, IgM and IgA, can be multimers of these), with differences in the heavy chains specifying the

Figure 7. Schematic of an IgG antibody

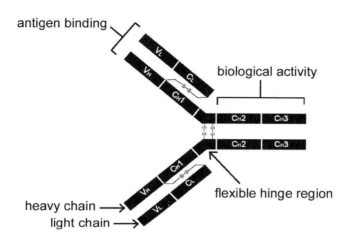

class to which the antibody belongs. Figure 7 shows a two dimensional model of the typical 4 chain structure of an IgG antibody. The heavy (H) and light (L) chains are made up of variable (V) and constant (C) region domains that have similar 3-dimensional structures. Note that the V regions of the H and L chains, which make up the antigen binding site, are on a different end of the molecule from the C regions, which are responsible for the biologic activity of the antibody. The identification of the 4 chain structure of antibodies was a tour-de-force of basic protein chemistry, and earned for Gerald Edelman and Rodney Porter the Nobel Prize in Medicine in 1972.

Antibodies are relatively stable proteins and can be modified for use in research or as diagnostic tools. Antibodies can be labeled with radioactive tracers such as ^{125}I, or covalently conjugated with biotin or fluorescent dyes, and still retain antigen specificity and biologic functions. Consequently, antibodies can be used to reveal the subcellular location of a protein, identify a protein band on a western blot, or identify a protein that binds a particular promoter sequence. They can be used to affinity purify a protein from a complex mixture of proteins, or be used to quantitate the levels of a hormone. The uses are limited only by the imagination of the investigator!

Nevertheless, polyclonal antibodies have one drawback: they must be continually produced by immunizing experimental animals and purified from their serum. This limits the amount of any antibody that can be isolated, and limits their distribution to other investigators, or their commercialization (although many polyclonal antibodies are produced for sale to the scientific community). This changed in 1975, when George Köhler

(1946–1995) and César Milstein (1927–2002) published their landmark paper in **Nature** describing *monoclonal antibody technology (29).*

B.　Monoclonal antibodies

Introduction

Monoclonal antibodies are antibodies derived from a clone of antibody producing cells that grow continuously in tissue culture and secrete antibodies of an identical and single specificity. The discovery of monoclonal antibody technology by Köhler and Milstein revolutionized biomedicine and has become a billion dollar industry. Remarkably, the inventors did not patent the technology, but their ingenious invention earned them the Nobel Prize in Medicine in 1984. Today, monoclonal antibodies are not only used as experimental tools by biomedical scientists, but as diagnostic tools in infectious disease, in screening for certain cancers, and as treatments for various diseases. Monoclonal antibody technology will continue to evolve for use in identifying disease markers and for use in fighting human diseases.

Production of monoclonal antibodies

The production of monoclonal antibodies relies on somatic cell genetic techniques. Somatic cell genetics involves the fusion of two different types of cells to produce a hybrid cell with one nucleus but with chromosomes contributed from both parental cells. In the case of antibody producing cells, Köhler and Milstein demonstrated that it was possible to immortalize cells producing antibodies of a desired specificity using somatic cell genetics by taking advantage of the indefinite growth characteristics of a particular type of tumor cell, a myeloma, and the antibody specificity of a B cell from an immunized animal.

The basic procedure for producing monoclonal antibodies is as follows. Spleen cells from immunized mice are isolated as a single cell suspension and fused to a myeloma cell line that grows in tissue culture. The fusion is now carried out using polyethylene glycol (PEG), although originally the Sendai virus, which fuses membranes, was used to facilitate fusion. The spleen cells (including the B cells) will die within a day or two in culture unless "rescued" by fusion with the myeloma. In turn, the myeloma cells that are used have been rendered defective in the enzyme hypoxanthine guanine phosphoribosyltransferase, or HGPRT, an enzyme involved in nucleic acid biosynthesis. These cells will die in tissue culture medium that is supplemented with hypoxanthine, aminopterin and thymidine (referred to as HAT medium) unless rescued by the HGPRT enzyme contributed by fused splenic B cells. Thus, only fused cells, called hybridomas, survive! The resulting hybridomas can be screened for the production of antibodies of the desired specificity. These can then be cloned to ensure that they are monoclonal and perpetuated indefinitely. A typical hybridoma produces one to several thousand antibody molecules per cell per second (!) and therefore can produce about 10^8 antibody molecules per day, which is about 25 picograms (pg; a pg is 10^{-12} g) of antibody. Using typical culture conditions, about 1 to 10 μg of antibody can be collected per ml of tissue culture medium, although systems have been developed that greatly improve the yield.

One other modification has been made to myeloma cells for the use in producing monoclonal antibodies. Myelomas are themselves malignantly transformed plasma cells and thus normally produce their own antibody molecules (usually of unknown specificity). Because the heavy and light chains of the myeloma antibodies can combine with the light and heavy chains of the antibodies contributed by the fused B cell, the original hybridomas produced "mixed antibodies" in addition to the antibodies of interest. Myelomas used today as fusion partners are those that have lost the ability to produce their own antibody molecules, although they retain the ability to secrete antibodies at high rates. The most widely used fusion partner is a myeloma referred to as SP2/0-Ag14, a myeloma derived from a tumor of a mouse.

Stable somatic fusions between cells can only be carried out using cells within a species or closely related species. Because the majority of myelomas that can be successfully adapted to tissue culture and be modified for use in producing hybridomas have come from mice, most moAb are derived from immunized rodents (mice, rats, and hamsters), although rabbit monoclonal antibodies have also been reported.

Humanized monoclonal antibodies

Antibodies from one species are themselves antigenic when injected into an unrelated species. Therefore, murine monoclonal antibodies that could otherwise be used for diagnostic purposes, or to attach a human tumor, cannot be safely administered more that once into humans without the potential for causing serious complications, including death. In fact, the danger in injecting antibodies from other species into humans was recognized in the first half of the 20th century, when the only treatment for tetanus infections (sometimes referred to as "lockjaw") was the administration of an anti-tetanus toxin to a patient produced in animals (usually horses). Tetanus is caused by bacterium *Clostridium tetani*, which releases a toxin that acts on nerves to cause muscle contractions that do not abate, and is often fatal. The administration of an anti-toxin

was often effective. However, while one treatment was generally toler-
ated by patients, a second injection often led to death, a reaction called
"serum sickness". Serum sickness is a hypersensitivity reaction with
symptoms similar to anaphylaxis that results from complications caused
by circulating soluble immune complexes formed between the infused
horse antibodies and the human anti-horse antibodies which deposit
into vital organs. As a result, a search for a source for human antibodies
against defined antigens has ensued.

However, no one has successfully developed a system to produce fully
human monoclonal antibodies with any reliability. Some human antibodies are produced by cells transformed by the Epstein Barr Virus (EBV,
the causative agent of mononucleosis) but these are not produced in
sufficient quantities to be particularly useful, and rarely have a desired
specificity. Consequently, mouse antibodies are often re-engineered by
recombinant DNA techniques to "humanize" the antibodies, with the goal
of retaining antigen specificity but otherwise being fully or near fully human in sequence. Therefore, sequences that encode the antigen binding
activity of the antibody are retained from the mouse sequence, but the
constant regions of the heavy and light chains and, in some cases the
"framework" regions within the variable region, those giving antibodies
their characteristic structure, are replaced with sequences common to
human antibodies. Humanized antibodies are much less immunogenic
than their mouse counterparts in humans and have longer half-lives
when injected. Some examples of humanized antibodies that have been
used in patients include Rituximab (Rituxin®), which is used in treating
B cell non-Hodgkins lymphoma, and Trastuzumab (Herceptin®), used
for treatment of metastatic breast cancer.

Phage display

Phage display is a method that incorporates the ability to genetically
manipulate bacteriophage and incorporate the gene elements encoding
the variable regions of an antibody molecule. The antibody gene segments are fused with the gene encoding the coat protein and thus the
antibodies are expressed in the phage. Phages can be produced with
a wide range of potential specificities using random sequences. Phage
with the desired specificity can then be isolated on the antigen, cloned,
and the V genes present identified for further use.

C.   Purification and use of antibodies

In order to obtain large quantities of polyclonal or monoclonal antibodies, it is often necessary to isolate them from serum or tissue culture

media, respectively. Although there are a number of methods that can be used, the most common is to take advantage of one of two bacterial proteins which bind antibodies (particularly IgG antibody classes) with high specificity. The antibodies can then be eluted (using low pH buffers) in pure form. These are protein A and protein G.

Protein A

Protein A is a cell wall constituent produced by the bacterium *Staphylococcus aureus* (the Cowan I strain is most commonly used). It is a protein of 42 kDa that binds to the Fc region of certain antibody molecules, specifically some of the IgG subclasses. The use of Protein A to purify IgG was introduced in 1975 (30). Protein A is used to detect or purify IgG or to isolate IgG-antigen complexes. It is often covalently bound to sepharose beads and can be reused a number of times due to its stability and resistance to denaturants.

Protein G

Protein G is a cell wall protein isolated from group G streptococci. It binds to IgG subclasses not recognized by protein A, and binds IgM antibodies as well. In its native form, protein G also binds albumin, Fab regions of antibodies, and constituents of cell membranes. To improve specificity, recombinant forms of protein G, in which only the Fc binding sites have been retained, have been produced and are now commercially available. Recombinant protein G is used in ways similar to protein A.

Antibodies as probes

The amazing versatility of antibodies is not only due to their remarkable variability and their high degree of specificity, but also due to the fact that the can be modified by covalent attachment of reagents that allow for their detection in a variety of assays. A few of the most common forms of modifications, and some of their uses, is listed below.

Iodinated antibodies

One of the first labeling techniques for antibodies was to covalently label them with a radioactive isotope of iodine, such as ^{125}I (^{131}I can also be used). Antibodies can be labeled to a high specific activity with ^{125}I without compromising antigen binding or biological activity. They can be used for both *in vivo* and *in vitro* studies. The use of radioactively-labeled antibodies was crucial to the development of the radioimmunoassay

(RIA; see below). The most common methods of iodination result in the chemical oxidation of Na^{125}I to reactive radioactive iodine using lactoperoxidase (an enzyme found in raw cow's milk) or chloramine-T (chloramines are compounds that are composed of chlorine and nitrogen and, interestingly, are widely used as antiseptics), which couple the ^{125}I to the phenyl side chains of tyrosine residues. Commercially prepared solid phase iodination reagents such as Pierce Biotechnology's "IODO-BEADS" are also often used.

Biotin-labeled antibodies

Biotin is one of the most commonly used reagents for generating non-radioactive probes. Biotin is a water soluble vitamin, vitamin H, a member of the vitamin B complex. The most visible sign of biotin-deficiency is thinning of the hair. Biotin can be covalently coupled to proteins, and covalently incorporated into DNA. Biotin is detected using avidin (an egg white protein) or streptavidin, both of which bind with high affinity. Streptavidin is a 60 kDa protein from the bacterium Streptomyces avidinii that has high affinity for biotin with a K_d (a measurement of the dissociation constant which is used to reflect the affinity of the interaction between two molecules) of 10^{-15}, orders of magnitude higher than most antibodies bind antigens. Streptavidin can be fluorescently labeled or conjugated with enzymes, such as alkaline phosphatase or horseradish peroxidase, and therefore can be used as a second-step reagent for the detection of biotinylated antibody or nucleic acid probes (in blotting reactions by chemiluminescence) or proteins detected by biotinylated antibodies by immunofluorescence. Streptavidin-coated beads are also used for affinity purification of biotinylated proteins or proteins bound to biotinylated antibodies.

Enzyme-linked antibodies

Enzymes such as horseradish peroxidase (HRP) and alkaline phosphatase (AP) can be covalently attached to antibodies to aid in their detection. Enzyme-linked antibodies are the reagents that make methods such as ELISA and immunohistochemistry possible (see below). For example, HRP (isolated from Amoracia rusticana, or horseradish root) combines with peroxide to oxidize a variety of substrates, and can be detected by the production of an insoluble product that is red-brown in color. Enzymes, especially HRP, are also the label of choice for Western blotting techniques using non-radioactive probes in which the bound antibodies are detected using enhanced chemiluminescence (ECL) to detect the enzyme linked antibody. Chemiluminescence is the direct transformation of chemical energy into light energy. For example, HRP oxidizes the substrate luminal (a chemical reaction) with the concomitant production of light, which is enhanced in the presence of a chemical enhancer. The light emission can be detected on photographic film or in chemiluminescent readers by digital cameras into a computer. While the dynamic range of film is between one and two orders of magnitude, chemiluminescent readers can detect and quantitated proteins over at least three orders of magnitude, and therefore provide more quantitative information.

Fluorescent antibodies

Antibodies can be covalently modified with a wide variety of fluorescent compounds. Albert Coons was the first to directly conjugate a fluorescent label to an antibody for visualization and demonstrate that the antibody still retained antigen binding activity (31). From this humble beginning, fluorescent antibodies have become one of the most useful reagents for study of basic questions in immunology, cell biology and neurobiology, and in clinical medicine. The power of techniques that utilize fluorescent antibodies and the advances they have made possible in biomedicine are underscored in subsequent sections devoted to these methods, and in Chapter 5. Today, there are a large number of different fluorescent molecules that have distinct excitation and emission spectra and can be applied to fluorescence microscopy and/or fluorescence activated cell sorting. These include fluorescein (FITC), Texas Red (TR), phycoerythrin (PE), allophycocyanin (APC), various "Cy dyes" (including Cy5, Cy7 etc.) and Alexa Fluor dyes (Alexa 488, Alexa 546, etc.), to name but a few. The Cy dyes and Alexa fluor dyes were designed to have higher intensities and reduced photobleaching properties than conventional fluors.

Colloidal gold labeling of antibodies

Antibodies can be labeled with colloidal gold beads of defined size to provide an electron dense tag which enables the use of antibodies in immunogold electron microscopy (Chapter 5) Gold beads of 5 nm, 10 nm and 15 nm are most commonly used. The colloidal gold interacts tightly with the antibody but is not covalently attached.

Methods to identify and quantitate antigens

Prior to the 1960s, the widespread use of antibodies was more qualitative than quantitative. Assays to measure antibody-antigen interactions relied on the ability of antibodies to cross-link soluble or cell-associated antigens, allowing for the detection of antigen-antibody interactions by agglutination reactions, or precipitation. Both methods rely on the fact that antibodies are multivalent (have two or more binding sites) and therefore can bind to epitopes on more than one cell, or more than one protein. As a result, antibodies that react with cells often cause the cells to be clumped together, the process known as agglutination. Agglutination is still the method used for ABO blood typing because it is inexpensive and rapid, and visible to the naked eye. When proteins (or other macromolecules) are cross-linked, they fall out of solution once the cross-linked matrix is of sufficiently large size, a process called immunoprecipitation. The precipitates can easily be large enough to be visible.

Immunoprecipitation

Immunoprecipitation is still widely used today to identify and biochemically characterize molecules from cells, cell extracts, or in vitro transcription-translation assays. Rather than relying on the antigen-antibody matrix to become large enough to precipitate on its own, however, protein A (or protein G) coupled to agarose or Sepharose beads is usually used to bring down the antigen-antibody complexes, which can then be processed for further analysis.

Radioimmunoassay (RIA)

The development of the RIA was a major breakthrough in the ability to rapidly and sensitively quantitate any biomolecule for which a antibody existed. As the name implies, the RIA is an immunoassay (a method of identifying and quantitating a substance using specific antibodies) that incorporates the use of a radioactively labeled ligand. It was developed by Yalow and Berson in 1959 and published a year later (32). The RIA permitted, for the first time, the determination of hormone levels in the blood (it was first developed for the measurement of insulin), and was rapidly adapted to a number of other research and clinical applications. The method is highly sensitive, and can detect antigens at concentrations of as little as a few pg. The development of this method earned for Rosalyn Yalow the Nobel Prize in Medicine in 1977.

The RIA is based on a competition assay in which a known amount of antibody is mixed with a known amount of radiolabeled antigen. Unlabeled antigen, often referred to as "cold" antigen, is then added to the mix in increasing concentrations, which displaces increased amounts of the labeled antigen, since the cold antigen "competes" for binding (much as in the same way that cold competitors compete for binding in EMSA; see Chapter 3). This allows for the establishment of a standard curve, in which the ratio of the bound antigen/free antigen is plotted versus the amount of unlabeled antigen added, where the bound/free is determined by counting the radioactivity associated with the antibody and that released from the antibody (there are a number of ways of separating these depending on how the assay is initially set up). By comparing the amount of radioactive antigen displaced by an "unknown" sample, the concentration of the antigen in the sample can be determined with accuracy.

Most radioimmunoassay employ the use of antigens labeled with radioactive iodine (^{125}I), but tritium (^{3}H)-labeled antigens are also sometimes used.

Enzyme-linked immunosorbent assay (ELISA)

The ELISA was first described by Engvall and Perlman in 1971 (33). ELISA is the most commonly used method for analysis of soluble antigens and antibodies. ELISA methods lend themselves to automation, making the quantitation of proteins in a large number of samples possible with relative ease. ELISAs are also highly sensitive, on par with RIA, do not involve the use of radioactivity, and can be used in a variety of permutations. In the most basic method, to quantitate an antibody response, wells of microtiter plates (96 well plates) are first coated with an antigen. Then serum samples (if an animal or person has been immunized) or supernatants (for example from tissue culture wells in which monoclonal antibodies are being screened) are added to the coated wells. After washing, a developing secondary antibody is added. Secondary antibodies are those that have been made in one species that recognize antibodies form a different species (for example, goat anti-mouse antibodies, or rabbit ant-goat antibodies, *etc.*) The secondary antibody is coupled to an enzyme (hence, the name "enzyme-inked"). The conversion of substrate is directly proportional to the amount of bound secondary antibody, which in turn is proportional to the amount of antibody bound to the antigen.

A second type of ELISA is the sandwich ELISA. In a sandwich ELISA, the plate is first coated with an antibody to the antigen, and the antigen added. This assay is particularly useful when pure forms of the antigen are not available. The remainder of the procedure is the same as outlined above. In general, sandwich ELISAs are the most sensitive and can detect proteins in concentrations of 100 pg/ml to 1 ng/ml (10^{-9} to 10^{-10} grams). Standard ELISAs are generally one order of magnitude less sensitive.

Enzyme-linked immunospot (ELISPOT) assays

The ELISPOT assay was originally developed as an alternative to the plaque assay (34) developed by Niels Jerne (who won the Nobel Prize for his theories on the specificity of the immune system in 1984). The plaque assay was developed as a method to detect and quantitate individual antibody secreting cells. This assay limited the range of antibody specificities that could be measured, and relied on an additional step of adding fresh serum (as a source of complement) to produce the characteristic plaques. The ELISPOT was developed to circumvent these issues. With improvements in the assay, it is now one of the two methods used to enumerate cytokine producing cells. A cytokine is a small protein molecule produced by cells of the immune system that regulates other immune cells. Many cytokines provide communication between the immune system and other cells of the body as well. With the use of high affinity antibodies, ELISPOT assays can detect cells that produce as few as 100 molecules of a protein per cell per second. Compare that with an antibody producing cell, which produces 1000 to 10,000 antibody molecules per cell per second.

The ELISPOT assay starts with a membrane (usually nitrocellulose) coated with a specific antibody against, for example, the cytokine of interest. The membrane is placed in microtiter wells. Cells are then added to the well and incubated overnight. A second antibody to the cytokine is added (coupled with an enzyme) and its presence is detected by addition of a substrate. The development of "spots" identifies the location of a single, cytokine producing cell.

FACS

FACS (see below) can also be used to identify cytokine producing cells. Cells are incubated to allow cytokine production as for ELISPOT. However, because FACS is a cell-based assay, an agent is added during incubation which allows cytokine production but prevents its secretion. Brefeldin A is commonly used for this purpose, which prevents forward trafficking and secretion of newly synthesized proteins. The cells can be permeabilized and stained with a fluorescenated anti-cytokine antibody.

D.   Flow cytometry and fluorescence activated cell sorting (FACS)

FACS is a method that allows the separation of different cell populations or organelles to be analyzed and isolated using fluorescently tagged antibodies. FACS was developed in the 1960's by Leonard A.

Hertzenberg from Stanford University. The first simple instrument could separate cells based on cell size, granularity, and one or two "colors" using different fluorescent tags. Today, with the advent of new fluorescent probes, three different fluorescent dyes can be used with a single laser (after the "compensation" is corrected for signal spillover between channels). FACS instruments are now routinely fitted with two lasers and are designed to separate cells based on eight or nine individual parameters using fluors with distinct excitation and emissions spectra. There are two functions of cell sorters, one to analyze subpopulations of cells, and the other to collect these different populations. The FACS is routinely used not only for basic scientific analysis in immunology and cell biology, but is also used for analysis of clinical specimens and for screening of novel monoclonal (including humanized) antibodies against various tissues, together with a host of other uses.

The FACS instrument basically has two types of detectors. The light detector is used to characterize cells that enter the analyzers by forward and side scatter. Forward and side scatter are used to discriminate between different types of cell populations in a mixed sample. Forward scatter provides information that can be used to determine the relative size of cells that are being analyzed through a FACS instrument. Side scatter provides information about the granularity of a population. Thus, for example, if white blood cells from the blood or spleen are analyzed through a FACS instrument, forward and side scatter can be used to identify the lymphocyte, monocyte, and macrophage populations and discriminate them from neutrophils and other granulocytes. In addition, photomultiplier tubes collect information based on the fluorescence emissions spectra of the cells that are being passaged through the instrument to determine what types of antibodies (and therefore what types of surface molecules) are present on individual cell populations. The excitation of the fluorescent tags is accomplished using one or more lasers that are capable of exciting fluors at different wavelengths.

Fluorescence labeling allows the identification of cells or organelles with different cell surface molecules. The FACS instrument can collect fluorescent signals in one of a number of different "channels" that correspond to different laser excitation and fluorescent emission wavelength. Cells can be analyzed at rates of 100,000 to 1,000,000 cells per minute (slower flow rates are generally required when sorting cells, see below). Fluorescence can be detected using antibodies in one of two ways. First, an antibody against a cell surface molecule can be conjugated with a fluorescent tag (direct immunofluorescence). Alternatively, an antibody against a cell surface marker can be utilized in an unconjugated form and detected using a secondary antibody, a method called indirect

Figure 8.   Fluorescence activated cell sorting plots

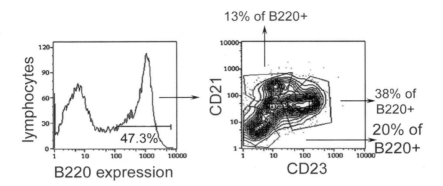

immunofluorescence. Both methods are highly sensitive and can detect as few as a few hundred to a thousand molecules on an individual cell.

Figure 8 shows one example of a FACS analysis. Spleen cells were run through a FACS analyzer and the lymphocyte gate was identified by forward and side scatter characteristics. The remainder of the analysis was performed on this isolated gate (by gating, you have the ability to exclude all other cells in a population from your analysis). The lymphocytes were stained with three different antibodies, each with a different fluorescent probe. The first detects B lymphocytes (B220) in the spleen cell populations (the other major type of lymphocyte is the T cell). The B220-positive B cells were then analyzed for the presence of two other cell surface molecules, CD21 and CD23, that can further divide B cells into functionally distinct populations (3 different populations are identified). Note two different types of FACS profiles are illustrated here. The left panel shows a histogram which discriminates between cells that highly express B220 and those that do not, while the right panel shows a contour plot in which cells are monitored by two different antibodies. The level of expression of a particular molecule is displayed on a log scale. Current FACS instruments can discriminate label intensities over a 4 log scale.

Using this type of an analysis, investigators can iteratively begin to identify smaller and smaller subsets of cells. With sophisticated instrumentation and accomplished users, investigators with the right collection of antibodies can isolate cells that are present at frequencies as low as 1 in 1,000 to 1 in 10,000 cells with high fidelity.

While the description so far deals with the analytical aspects of a FACS instrument, FACS analysis is coupled with cell sorting technology that allows an investigator to isolate individual populations of cells. Therefore, the investigator can instruct the FACS to collect individual populations of cells and put them in individual tubes or even put single cells with the desired phenotype in individual wells of a 96-well microtiter plate. This allows for rapid cloning of cells as well as for study of subpopulations under defined *in vitro* conditions. FACS can also be used to isolate and study distinct subtypes of cells in certain tumors, *etc*.

It should be noted that while most FACS staining is performed on intact cells, intracellular proteins can also be evaluated using FACS by first fixing and permeabilizing the cells. Common agents for permeabilization are discussed in Chapter 5.

In addition to analyzing and isolating cells based on cell surface characteristics, FACS can be used for studying a number of other cell characteristics. Some of these are briefly outlined below.

DNA content and cell cycle analysis

Propidium iodide (PI), DAPI (4',6'-diamidino-2-phenylindole hydrochloride) and Hoechst dyes bind to DNA and become fluorescent. Because these dyes bind DNA stoichiometrically, they can be used to analyze DNA content and also provide cell cycle information. DNA staining can be used to study cell cycle since relative DNA content can show the proportion of cells in G1, G2 and S phases of the cell cycle. Neither PI nor DAPI enter live cells, but some of the Hoechst dyes do, and therefore the analysis is generally performed after cell fixation or permeabilization. In addition, cells undergoing apoptosis can be discriminated from live cells based on their forward and side scatter characteristics as well as DNA characteristics.

Apoptosis

Apoptosis, or programmed cell death, is one of two major types of cell death. Apoptosis can be distinguished from necrotic death by a number of characteristic properties of the apoptotic cells. The FACS can be used to identify the cells in several different ways.

Annexin V

Annexin V is a member of a calcium and phospholipid binding family of proteins that binds to phosphatidyl serine. Phosphatidyl serine is usually on the inner leaflet of the plasma membrane but is exposed on the surface of apoptotic cells. When the Annexin V is fluoresceinated and used in combination with PI, the apoptotic cells can be discriminated on the basis of low PI staining and high Annexin V fluorescence.

TUNEL assay

TUNEL (terminal deoxynucleotidyl transferase mediated dUTP nick-end labeling) is a sensitive method to identify apoptotic cells. During apoptosis, nonrandom DNA fragmentation occurs, and the enzyme TdT and can be used to attach labeled dUTP to the 3'-hydroxyl DNA ends of the fragmented DNA. The dUTP can be labeled with a variety of tags, including fluorescent markers or with biotin. The number of cells with fragmented DNA can be determined using FACS, but this method works equally well with tissue sections and adherent cells.

Of course, there are non-FACS-based methods for analyzing apoptosis. The DNA from cells that are undergoing apoptosis also give a characteristic laddering due to nonrandom fragmentation, and this can be viewed on agarose gels (using ethidium bromide stained DNA).

Miscellaneous FACS based assays

Calcium flux

One of the earliest signals in cells when ligand binds the receptor is often a flux in cellular calcium. FACS can be used to monitor calcium fluxes upon ligand receptor interactions. Calcium flux is frequently measured using Indo-1. Because INDO-1 has a different fluorescence emissions spectra when it is bound to calcium and when it is not, an increase in cellular calcium will result in a rapid increase in fluorescence intensity.

Cell proliferation

Cell proliferation can be monitored in cells that have been stained with the dye CFSE (carboxy-fluorescein diacetate, succinimidyl ester). CSFE contains a fluorescein molecule and diffuses freely into cells. Intracellular esterases cleave acetate groups on the CSFE which converts it into a fluorescent, membrane-impermeant dye. The dye remains in the cells and is not transferred, nor does it (to anyone's knowledge) adversely affect cellular functions. During each round of cell division, the relative intensity of the dye is decreased by half, therefore, one can monitor the number of cell divisions that an individual cell or population of cells is going through by monitoring the decreased levels of CSFE in the individual cells up to 3–4 cell divisions.

Gene expression studies

FACS is frequently used to identify cells that have activated the reporter gene (for example, in promoter constructs that use GFP, or in constructs that have a particular gene that is fused "in-frame" with the GFP so that a chimeric protein is expressed. Cells that contain the GFP can be distinguished from those that do not because of the fluorescent properties of the protein, making GFP a convenient marker for gene expression to discriminate transfected from untransfected cells.

E.   Other assays using antibodies

Immunohistochemistry (IH or IHC)

Immunohistochemistry is a method that allows for the localization of antigens in tissue sections using specific antibodies. IH is sometimes referred to as immunocytochemistry (localization of antigens in cells, rather than tissues) or immunostaining. The reactions between the antibodies and the antigens in the tissues are most often revealed by enzymatic reactions (much like western blotting or ELISA) or using fluorescence, and thus can be visualized under a light or fluorescent microscope. However, radioactive or colloidal gold-labeled antibodies can also be used for IH, the latter for EM immunohistochemistry.

The first use of an antibody for IH was reported in 1942 by A. Coons, who used a fluorescent antibody to reveal antigen distribution in a tissue section (35). Since then, many improvements in the methods for tissue harvest and sectioning and the preparation of the tissue for antibody staining have improved. Most IH is performed using flash-frozen tissue (using liquid nitrogen, which has a temperature of $-196°C$, or $-320°F$) that is sectioned using cryostats, which allows for preservation of the original tissue architecture and antigenic structures. IH is an invaluable tool for studying the basic architecture and cellular localization in tissues, changes that occur during disease states, and for diagnostic purposes.

Surface plasmon resonance

Surface plasmon resonance is an extremely sensitive method for determining the concentration and affinities of the interactions between antibodies and antigens, or between receptors and their ligands. Surface plasmon resonance is the response measured when light is reflected under defined conditions from a conducting film (usually a gold film) that interfaces two media with different refractive indexes. The sensor surface is coated with a receptor (or antibody). After addition of the ligand, the response (as resonance units) is measured using very specialized instrumentation. The RU can be converted concentration of the ligand on the sensor surface, and the affinities determined. Surface plasmon resonance is sensitive to changes as little as a pg/mm^2 on the sensor.

Chapter 5

MICROSCOPY: IMAGING OF BIOLOGICAL SPECIMENS

A.   Introduction

Imaging technologies seek to peer inside tissues, cells, or even an entire organism, including man, to reveal underlying structures. The most common methods of imaging use the microscope. The use of microscopes has become an essential part of almost every field of biomedical sciences, and is particularly important in the field of Cell Biology, which seeks to understand how cells are organized and function.

Anton van Leeuwenhoek of Holland is generally considered to be the father of the microscope. The first "light microscope" was invented by him in the mid 17th century. Convex lenses, the essential component required for magnification, had been developed about 100 years earlier. The single lens design limited the amount of magnification possible. The development of the compound microscope late in the 17th century helped overcome this limitation. A compound microscope is a microscope consisting of 2 lenses, one the "objective" and the second the "eyepiece". It was with these early microscopes that the Englishman Robert Hooke looked at the unseen world and gave the name "cell" to describe the smallest observable structures that made up living organisms. Later, Louis Pasteur was able to identify yeast organisms, and Robert Koch discovered the bacilli (rod shaped bacteria) that cause tuberculosis *(Mycobacterium tuberculosis)* and cholera *(Vibrio cholerae)*. Real changes in microscope design did not occur until the 19th century when Carl Zeiss, the founder of the microscope company, began to standardize compound microscope design and engaged experts in optics to improve the quality of the lenses used in microscopes. These designs helped push the light microscope to the limits of its capabilities.

The development of the electron microscope by Max Knoll and Ernst Ruska in Germany in the early 1930's was the first truly significant

Table 4. Selected Nobel Laureates *(Cell Biology and Imaging)*

Camillo Golgi Santiago Ramón y Cajal	structure of cells of the nervous system	1906[†]
Albert Claude Christian de Duve George E. Palade	application of microscopy and differential centrifugation to elucidate structure of the cell	1974[†]
Nicolaas Bloembergen Arthur Leonard Schawlow Kai M. Siegbahn	development of lasers; electron spectroscopy	1981[‡]
Aaron Klug	adaptation of EM and structural modeling to viruses and nucleic acid-protein interactions	1982[*]
Ernst Ruska Gerd Binnig Heinrich Rohrer	designs of first electron microscope and scanning tunneling microscope	1986[‡]
Paul C. Lauterbur Sir Peter Mansfield	development of magnetic resonance imaging	2003[†]

[†]Nobel Prize in Physiology or Medicine
[‡]Nobel Prize in Physics
[*]Nobel Prize in Chemistry

advance in microscope design since the construction of compound microscopes. The transmission electron microscope allowed scientists not only to look at the surface, but to peer inside, living cells and discover their complexity. It allowed us to see viruses for the very first time, and it also made it possible to look at cell membranes, and even some large protein complexes. Ernst Ruska was award the Nobel Prize in 1986 for the development of the transmission electron microscope, a prize he shared with two scientists, Heinrich Rohrer and Gerd Binnig, for their development of the scanning tunneling microscope (Table 4), which is used to study atoms on physical surfaces, such as silicon chips for computers. However, because samples that are being visualized in an electron microscope must be maintained in a vacuum, this technology does not allow cell biologist to study details of living cells.

The advent of fluorescent microscopic techniques by Albert H. Coons, using "labeled" antibodies and other probes to directly visualize tissues and components cells, and the coupling of the microscope to high resolution digital cameras and the computer, has truly revolutionized the use of microscope. Not only does direct transfer of images from a digital still or movie camera into a microscope allow an investigator to capture and store data, but it has promoted the development of sophisticated imaging software as well. Such software programs allow images to be significantly enhanced, extending the resolution of the light microscope. It is now possible to look within live cells and document the movements of their very dynamic structural components, the organelles, or to look within tissues and observe living cells moving within them. The addition of motorized stages or objectives on the microscope now allows investigators to look not only at a flat image of a cell, but to progressively "slice through" the cell from bottom to top. Thus, cells can be visualized not only in two dimensions, but in three dimensions. The capture of the information from the third dimension, the so-called z-stack, once rendered by computational software within the computer, now allows for the reconstruction of a three-dimensional image of the cell. Together with conventional biochemical techniques, a much deeper understanding of cell structure and function is emerging from the use of modern light microscopes.

The following sections outline some of the methodology that is used to image cells and tissues at high resolution.

B.   Light microscopy

Light microscopy is a generic term for a variety of techniques that all employ a standard compound microscope. Specimens are usually placed on slides for viewing, and may be living or fixed (and therefore are not viable). Some microscopes are fitted with stage adaptors that keep samples warmed to biological temperatures. This allows the activity of the cells, or organelles within them, to be viewed over time using time-lapse photography.

Phase-contrast

The simplest form of light microscopy uses "brightfield" illumination, in which a beam of light is focused on the object to be viewed. Although cells and tissues can be seen, many biological specimens are almost transparent under these conditions. Consequently, contrast is poor, and details are lacking. Phase-contrast helps to correct this by improving the resolution of unstained biological specimens. This method was adapted in the late 1930's and 1940's by Zeiss laboratories. The contrast of cells is improved because the image is revealed as lighter or darker depending on the different densities within the cell being viewed; the greater the density, the longer the path length of the light being viewed, and therefore the darker they appear.

Differential interference contrast (DIC)

DIC microscopy, also known as **Nomarski optics**, is a method used to further increase the surface contrast of specimens in greater detail than is possible with phase contrast. DIC uses prisms to split light; when the light recombines in a second prism, any differences in surface topology will be reflected in an altered optical path, resulting in increased contrast. The method produces monochromatic shadowed images where optical path length gradients are introduced, which produces superior contrast into the images.

C.   Fluorescence and laser confocal microarray microscopy

Introduction to standard (widefield) fluorescence microscopy

Fluorescence microscopy takes advantage of fluorescently labeled "probes" to visualize the location of a target molecule within cells or tissues. Rather than visualizing the specimen itself, fluorescent microscopes reveal the localization of a target molecule by illuminating the fluorescent probe. These probes are usually antibodies (polyclonal or monoclonal) or lectins (proteins that bind specific sugar residues), and may be directly labeled with a fluor, or themselves specifically detected with a secondary reagent that is labeled. Most fluorescent microscopes use "epifluorescence", meaning that the excitatory light is transmitted through the objectives onto the specimen and not through the specimen. In this way, only the reflected excitatory light needs to be filtered, which reduces "noise" in the signal.

Fluorescent molecules

Fluorescent molecules absorb light of a particular wavelength and emit it at longer wavelengths. Fluorescent microscopes pass light through "excitation" and "emission" filters that allow the visualization of the fluorescent probe. A variety of probes that emit at different wavelengths are now available. This allows investigators to sequentially visualize a number of different target molecules within regions of the cell, yielding a variety of colors including greens, reds, yellows, blues, etc. This not only has greatly enhanced the ability of cell biologists to visualize the localization and movement of proteins and organelles within cells, but the pictures can have the most amazing "wow" effect! Fluorescence microscopy is used to characterize the organization of cells, and the compartments within cells (nucleus, Golgi, endoplasmic reticulum, plasma membrane and endosomal compartments, etc.), as well as the vesicles and tubules that transport "cargo" between these compartments. In order to label intracellular proteins with specific antibodies, the cells must first be fixed and permeabilized so that the antibodies can gain entry to the cell. Common fixation agents include paraformaldehyde and formaldehyde. Permeabilization of aldehyde-fixed cells is usually accomplished with a detergent, such as Triton X-100 or saponin at very low concentrations, lower than would normally be used to solubilize cells. The agents that are used for fixation and permeabilization are strictly cell and antibody dependent. Methanol can be used as both a fixative, which also permeabilizes the cell. Finally, in some (rare) cases, permeabilization without fixation can be accomplished with pore-forming agents such as streptolysin-O (SLO). SLO is a toxin that comes from Streptococcus aureus. It binds cholesterol in membranes and aggregates, forming pores. SLO is used more often as a means to deplete cells of cytosolic contents in systems that strive to define the cytosolic requirements for intracellular vesicular trafficking by reconstitution.

Fixation and permeabilization of cells, also kills them cell, so that the localization of target molecules are frozen in time. However, the localization and movement of molecules can be visualized using chimeric proteins, expressing variants of the green fluorescent protein (GFP) or its spectral variants, such as YFP and CFP. Indeed, YFP and CFP are the most common tags used for FRET analysis (see below).

Fluorescent microscopy can be combined with other methods that are used to enhance contrast in cells, such as phase contrast and DIC. These methods can be used to first localize the specimen on the slide, since the illuminating light does not photobleach the probe, which degrades the sensitivity of the assay. In addition, contrast imaging and fluorescent images can be superimposed in a single image to reveal both the entire cell or tissue and the fluorescent probes.

There are limitations to standard fluorescence microscopy. The first is the "out of focus spreading" that occurs when the entire specimen is illuminated, even though the microscope is focused only on one plane of the cell. This gives significant background and can frequently impair resolution of internal structures. Second, the probes in the out of focus areas, because they are illuminated, photobleach, resulting in degradation of the intensity of staining. To overcome these problems, other methods have been developed to visualize fluorescent probes in individual planes of biological samples with high sensitivity and resolution.

Laser confocal microscopy

Confocal microscopy is an optical sectioning method that selectively collects images from a selected focal plane using a directed beam of light from a laser. In a confocal microscope, the depth of the optical sections

Figure 9.   Comparison of immunofluorescence and laser confocal microscopy

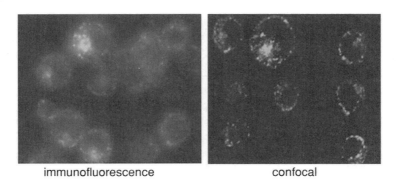

immunofluorescence   confocal

can be controlled, but generally sections of 0.8 μm are collected. These sections are sufficient to resolve organelles at relatively high resolution, but are too thick for details on vesicular compartments within the cell. The design of the confocal microscope evolved over a period of 8 to 10 years to the type of system used today (reviewed in 36). The functionality of confocal microscopy is dependent on computer software for collecting images from the microscope. The key advantage of confocal microscopy is that filtering is used to eliminate out-of-focus signals that otherwise degrades the quality of the image created in standard wide-field fluorescent microscopy. Figure 9 shows two fluorescent images of B lymphocytes, one collected using standard immunofluorescence, the other using laser confocal microscopy. Note the clarity of the confocal image, while the image that is collected using a standard fluorescence microscope is hazy due to the out of focus fluorescence. Only one probe is used for these images: image the difference in clarity when 3 or 4 different fluorescent probes are combined to localize different proteins and compartments within a single cell!

Because optical sections can be collected, a major advantage of confocal microscopy is that serial optical sections (in the X-Y plane) can be collected. As a result, confocal microscopy not only provides information on structures in an individual plane, but can collect multiple sections in the z direction, generating a z-stack. Computer programs can then reconstruct an optical image of the cell in 3-dimensions.

There are disadvantages of laser confocal microscopy. First, while the optical sectioning rejects out-of-focus light, the laser generates fluorescence even in these out-of-focus planes. This results in photobleaching of the non-imaged areas of the cells and, consequently, significantly brighter images are required for confocal microscopy than standard immunofluorescence. As a result, confocal microscopy is less than optimal for resolving proteins that are expressed at relatively low abundance.

Two-photon excitation microscopy

Two photon microscopy is used for imaging relatively thick tissue samples rather than individual cells. It allows for the collection of a 3-dimensional image of a section with absorption of light either above or below the focal plane, and therefore there is little photobleaching of the out-of-focus images within the sample. Two photon microscopy allows for the imaging of events at some distance from the surface of tissues and has been used to examine intact viable tissues, therefore providing the opportunity to visualize cell organization and movement within a live tissue.

Two-photon microscopy is based on the principle that fluorophores that can be excited at a particular wavelength can also be excited by two red photons at twice the wavelength. High energy lasers are needed to generate the energy required for this type of microscopy.

Deconvolution Microscopy

Deconvolution microscopy is computationally intense image process-ing technique that can be used to generate optically sectioned images from standard widefield fluorescent microscopy (37). Its advantage over laser confocal microscopy is that it can be used to collect images at lower light than using confocal microscopy, and it does not result in the intense photobleaching common with confocal beams. Deconvolution acquires images from multiple focal planes in the cell and uses iterative mathematical algorithms to reassign the light to its original fluorescent source. The resulting image (on the computer, not in the microscope!) is an accurate rendering of the cell which can be viewed as a single focal plane or as a 3-dimensional structure, similar to images generated by confocal microscopy.

Total internal reflection (TIR) fluorescence microscopy

TIR fluorescence microscopy is a method that can be used to analyze events that occur just below the plasma membrane of a cell, to a depth of approximately 50 nm. It is often used to visualize the docking and fusion of secretory vesicles to the plasma membrane. TIR functions by reducing the background fluorescence within the cell. In standard epifluorescence, the excitation light beam shines directly on the sample at a 90° angle. In TIR, the light is focused through a prism into the glass coverslip so that the sample is struck by the beam at a shallow angel (23°). Consequently, only fluorophores near the plasma membrane are excited by the light, rather than the bulk of the cellular material. The rest is physics and math. However, TIR is the only fluorescent microscopy method that allows some detailed insights into endocytic and exocytic events at the cell surface.

Fluorescence resonance energy transfer (FRET)

Fret is a method that allows for the identification of proteins that interact within live cells, either stably or transiently. FRET requires the expression of two different interacting proteins in a cell that are each labeled with distinct fluorescent molecules that are capable of transferring energy. In FRET, the exited fluorophore (the donor) transfers energy to a second longer wavelength fluorophore (the acceptor). Note that the transfer can also be considered a quenching reaction because there is no emission of fluorescence by the donor fluorophore. As outlined in Chapter 3, FRET is also used in real-time PCR.

In general, the proteins to be studied using FRET are genetically modified as fusion proteins to contain one of two different green fluorescent protein derivatives, CFP and YFP (see Chapter 4 for more information). FRET is highly sensitive to the distance between the two labeled proteins, requiring that they be within 10 nm (or 100 Å) before energy transfer can take place. The interaction of the two proteins results in energy transfer, which is detected by computer-based software that receives signals from digital cameras on the microscope. Because it is a microscopic method, FRET provides direct insights into the intracellular compartment(s) in which protein-protein interactions occur.

Fluorescence recovery after photobleaching (FRAP)

FRAP is a live cell imaging technique that is used to study the movement and redistribution of fluorescent molecules. Most experiments now take advantage of chimeric proteins with in-frame GFP or one of its variants. In a FRAP experiment, a portion of the cell is exposed to a high intensity light from a laser to irreversibly photobleach fluorescent proteins within a discrete region of the cell. The recovery of fluorescence in the same region therefore is due to the migration of fluorescent molecules from other areas of the cell into the photobleached region. FRAP has been used to study protein mobility and dynamics in a number of cellular compartments, including the endoplasmic reticulum, Golgi, and plasma membrane.

D. Electron Microscopy (EM)

Introduction

No matter how sophisticated the microscope or the software used to resolve the images, light microscopes are limited by the physics of light: objects less than 200 nm (0.2 μm) in size simply cannot be resolved, although smaller images can be identified by fluorescent signals using fluorescent microscopy. This limitation helped drive the development of the electron microscope in the 1930s (38), which can magnify objects >300,000 times, and can resolve objects of a nm or less in size! Instead of using light, electron microscopes use electrons as a source for imaging. Ernst Ruska won the Nobel Prize in Physics in 1986 for the development of the electron microscope, 4 years after chemist Aaron Klug won the Nobel Prize for adapting the use of EM to help determine the structure of nucleic acid-protein complexes in biologically relevant organisms, especially viruses. One of Klug's earliest studies using EM was published in 1964 (39).

Electrons are affected by any matter that they encounter, including air. As a result, samples to be imaged in an electron microscope must be kept in a vacuum. Consequently, live samples cannot be resolved! In addition, a variety of methods must be employed to provide contrast to biological membranes so that the object that is being resolved can actually be seen.

Transmission electron microscope (TEM)

The TEM images electrons that pass through a sample, and can therefore visualize internal structures of cells and tissues. In TEM, the electrons that pass through a sample are imaged; therefore, the darker areas that are visualized from a phosphor image screen are the thicker and denser areas, which allow fewer electrons to pass through.

For conventional TEM, sample specimens must be cut very thin and should be dry (water is opaque to electrons). Because biological samples are primarily water, the water must be removed from the sample, and the sample prepared so that they diffract electrons, which they do not do naturally. Preparing samples for TEM that retain "native" structural morphology is a challenge that many consider an art form. A number of protocols have been developed for this purpose of the past decades, a few of which are mentioned below.

Ultrathin sectioning and plastic embedding

This is one of the most frequently used methods for examining biological samples. Fixed samples are stained with heavy metals, usually osmium tetroxide and uranyl acetate, dehydrated with ethanol or acetone to remove water, and embedded in plastic for sectioning. Because harsh chemicals are used prior to embedding, antigenic structures are often not retained, and therefore antibodies cannot be combined with plastic embedding procedures.

Immunogold electron microscopy

To detect antigenic structures within cells and tissues using TEM, samples are more carefully protected prior to sectioning. The samples are cryo-protected with agents such as sucrose and flash frozen in liquid nitrogen, which protects the organization of the subcellular structures. Cryosectioning is then carried out at temperatures as low as −120°C using an ultramicrotome. Ultramicrotomes are generally fitted with diamond-edged knives and are able to cut sections as thin as 60 nm. Antibodies that are labeled with colloidal gold particles (see Chapter 4) can be added in order to specifically identify the localization of protein antigens found within intracellular compartments. Contrast is provided by staining sections with agents such as uranyl acetate, dried and examined by TEM. Figure 10 shows an immunogold labeled-section of a plasma cell that is labeled with an antibody against the IgM antibody that is being synthesized and secreted by the cell. The section shown demonstrates the presence of high concentrations of the newly synthesized IgM antibody (denoted by the electron dense colloidal gold on the anti-IgM antibody) within the endoplasmic reticulum of the cell (the narrow, membrane contained organelle).

Figure 10. Immunogold electron microscopy

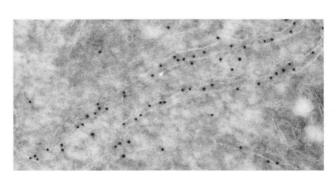

Negative staining

While the addition of heavy metals can be used to provide contrast to intracellular organelles, these positive staining methods do not always provide the best contrast for surface structures, such as the plasma membrane. For this purpose negative staining procedures are often employed. These involve the embedding of cells or other particles, such as viruses, in metals that provide contrast. Because the biologic sample is less dense than its surroundings, this method is referred to as "negative" staining.

Freeze-fracture and deep etching

This method has been developed to allow for a very high resolution 3-dimensional image to be obtained of a sample, both of surface and internal structures. It incorporates a method known as rotary shadowing. In freeze-fracture, a "replica" is made of a sample, and this rather than the sample, is examined by TEM. The sample is frozen and fractured while under vacuum. The sample is "etched" by allowing it to dehydrate under vacuum (some techniques expose samples to extensive freeze drying, which leads to "deep etching"), and then a replica is made using a thin coating of a heavy metal such as platinum (the shadowing), which is then coated with carbon. Using this method, the thickness of the accumulated metal varies with the surface topography, and very high resolution images, with a 3-dimensional effect, is revealed.

Variations on TEM

A wide variety of methods has been and continues to be developed to improve the capabilities of TEM. For example, new mixed procedures, such as correlative video light electron microscopy, combine fluorescent microscopy and TEM for analyzing dynamic structures within cells. Cells expressing a fluorescent reporter such as GFP can be monitored by fluorescence, and then analyzed by TEM after fixation. Three-dimensional reconstructive methods are then used to overlay the two images.

Scanning electron microscope (SEM)

SEM was developed in 1942 but was not commercialized until the 1960s. The SEM (NOT to be confused with a scanning tunneling electron microscope; Table 4) is capable of imaging electrons emitted from a sample, and therefore is used to study surface structures. It uses lenses to focus a magnetized electron beam at a surface, and the interactions of the beam with the surface results in signals that have different energies and properties. This translates into a significant "depth of field" which is not possible with TEM. SEM can have resolutions of a few nm, and are generally used to identify surface features and topography of cells and tissues.

E.   Magnetic resonance imaging (MRI)

MRI is a non-invasive method for imaging tissues in 3 dimensions in living subjects. It is used for a variety of medical purposes, such as identifying solid and metastatic tumors, evaluating joint structure in individuals with autoimmune diseases or sports related injuries, or examining blood flow in the brain, *etc*. The development of MRI revolutionized diagnostic medicine, since many things that were only revealed in the past by exploratory surgery can now be imaged in a non-invasive, completely harmless manner. In addition to diagnostics, the MRI is also used as a powerful research tool. For example, functional MRI can be used to compare blood flow and brain functioning in normal subjects compared with patients with various forms of dementia, including Alzheimer's disease, as a means to identify and understand changes that may occur during the development of these diseases. For their roles in the development of MRI technology, Paul Lauterbur and Peter Mansfield were awarded the Nobel Prize in Medicine in 2003.

The design for the MRI developed by Lauterbur and Mansfield was directly applicable to human studies and diagnostics, and proved to be a very workable and adaptable MRI system. However, it was not the first MRI design. The first prototypic MRI instrument and patents were developed by Raymond Damadian, who published his work in 1971 (40), 2 years before Lauterbur (41) and Mansfield (42) published their first papers. Consequently, when the Nobel Prize for the MRI was announced, it generated an unusual amount of controversy, more so than normally accompany a Nobel Prize. It was the public nature of the controversy that set this Nobel Prize apart from others. Full page advertisements protesting the decision were taken out on behalf of Damadian, but to no avail.

MRI is based on principles similar to NMR (see Chapter 1). The sample (i.e., person) is placed within a strong magnetic field, and a radiofrequency field is then passed through the sample at a 90° angel to the magnetic field. The energy of the protons is increased when they absorb radio energy of the frequency. Radio waves are emitted by the atomic nuclei when they return to their previous energy level. Paul Lauterbur realized that by introducing gradients to the magnetic fields that were used for MRI, the source of the emitted waves could be traced, resulting in a two dimensional view of the structures emitting the radio waves. Peter Mansfield developed the methods for mathematical analysis of the waves, making imaging a real possibility. Today, the emitted waves are translated by the computers in the MRI into a 3-dimensional image. MRI works well in imaging because 70% of the body is comprised of water, and (as discussed in Chapter 1) hydrogen is the only natural atom that responds to NMR. Because the content of water varies significantly between soft tissues and bone, so do the proton concentrations, which gives sharp contrast between these tissues.

Within the soft tissues of the body, the differences are more subtle. New contrast agents have been developed that selectively enhance the images from different tissues. It has been said that as fluorescent probes made possible optical imaging, that MRI contrast agents have done the same for MRI, improving resolution to near cellular levels (as little as 10 μm)! Today, MRI is a standard tool in diagnosis: by the end of 2002, 60 million MRI images had already been taken!

Chapter 6

THE DERIVATION AND MANIPULATION OF EXPERIMENTAL ANIMALS IN BIOMEDICAL SCIENCES

A.   Introduction

Scientists strive to perform as many experiments as possible *in vitro*, using defined cell lines, isolated proteins, and their cloned counterparts. *In vitro* experiments have many advantages, including the ability to use purified reagents under controlled conditions so that other variables that could affect the experimental outcome are eliminated. However, the test tube is not a replacement for the complex interactions that occur in living organisms, and cell lines cannot replicate the alterations that arise during a disease state. Consequently, the use of experimental animals is a necessary, *albeit* controversial, component of biomedical research.

Experimental animals are an invaluable resource for mapping and identifying genes that contribute to disease susceptibility, for testing the functions of normal genes and their mutant counterparts in context, and for the testing of drugs to treat a variety of diseases. A few animal species have proven most useful because their genetic makeup can be altered either by controlled breeding or by experimental manipulation. Experimentally, it is now possible to introduce new genes into the genomes of these animals. It is also possible to "target" existing genes and mutate them, or delete them altogether. These animals, primarily rodent species, have proven especially helpful as the genes that cause human diseases have been mapped, and their identity determined. Animal studies have allowed scientists to both determine the normal functions of these genes, and to establish high fidelity animal models of human diseases for study and for testing new therapies for the treatment of these diseases. Genetically altered rodents, especially mice, are used to study the affects of genes and gene products in essentially all fields in biomedical science, from genetics to cell biology, neurobiology to cancer biology, and immunology to developmental biology.

So, what makes us so sure we can extrapolate from studies in mice any information that is applicable to humans? There are several reasons. First, the number of nucleotides in rodents and humans, and indeed in all mammalian species, is roughly the same, about 3 billion bp. Second, the number of genes in these species is the same, and by and large (with only a few exceptions) there is a 1:1 relationship between a gene in a human and in the mouse. Thus, for any given gene in the human genome there is a counterpart with a similar if not identical function in the mouse. Third, and more remarkably, the location and linkages of genes on the chromosomes is very similar. Thus, by mapping a disease susceptibility gene in the mouse, investigators already may have insights into where to search, and what to search for, in humans. True, mouse and human genes differ in nucleotide sequence, with an average difference of 20% to 30% per gene, but some are very conserved.

In this section, some of the methods used to alter the genetic makeup of mice, by both breeding and experimental manipulation, will be presented.

B.   Inbred strains of mice

At the beginning of the 20th century, scientists were attempting to develop ways to study the characteristics of tumors. They could readily identify cancers that would spontaneously develop in experimental animals, but because tissue culture techniques had not been developed, there was no way to propagate these cells *in vitro*. As an alternative approach, investigators attempted to passage (transfer) these tumors from one experimental animal to another, but they invariably failed to grow. Today we understand that these tumors were rejected by the immune response of the recipient animal against the histocompatibility antigens expressed on the tumor, much like transplanted organs between two unrelated persons are rejected.

A breakthrough in the ability to study tumors occurred when scientists used transplanted tumors that spontaneously arose within closed colonies of mice. These were mice that had been bred for certain rare characteristics. In the 18th, 19th, and early 20th centuries, the collecting of mice with unusual features was a popular hobby, and mouse fanciers around the world were always on the lookout for such mice. Two of the most collectable mice were albino mice (which are white and have pink eyes due to lack of pigmentation) and "Japanese Waltzing" mice. Japanese Waltzing mice could not stand up straight, but would turn in circles, and lose their balance. This characteristic is now known to be caused by an inner ear defect. In both cases, the mice were maintained by mouse breeders in closed colonies in order to maintain these interesting mutations, which were known to be recessive traits. Cancer biologists soon found that if they took a tumor that spontaneously arose in one member of these closed colonies that they could often successfully transplant them to another member of the colony. The tumor would grow in this mouse, and thus the investigator had a near perpetual source of a singe type of tumor for study. This led to the development of inbreeding of mice to generate genetically identical animals for experimental use.

Inbreeding is nothing more than a tool to restrict heterozygosity in an animal. Most animals cannot be inbred because they fix deleterious recessive mutations which are generally lethal. However, inbred lines have been generated in a small number of experimental animals, including mice, rats, guinea pigs, and even rabbits. Mice are by far the easiest species in which to establish inbred strains. Inbreeding is usually carried out by continual brother/sister mating. Each generation, a single male and female offspring of a mating is selected for breeding. When this has been accomplished through 20 generations (luckily, the gestation time for mice is relatively short so that this can be accomplished within an investigator's lifetime!), an inbred strain has been developed. Statistically, this leads to animals that are greater than 99.999% identical, one to another, the "identical twins" of the mouse world. To be sure that the animals are genetically pure, breeding laboratories will continue inbreeding the animals.

Many inbred strains of mice are named after their originator or to identify the characteristics that were selected during the inbreeding. For example, BALB/c mice, an albino strain, is named after the Ohio mouse dealer from which the breeding stock was obtained (Halsey Bagg's ALBino; the "c" is the gene symbol for albinism). The DBA strain of mice is named for three recessive genes that influence coat color in mice, dilute, brown, and non-agouti and, in fact, was the first inbred strain produced. C57BL and C57BR mice were derived from female mouse # 57 from the colony of a mouse breeder, "Miss Abbey Lathrop", in Granby, Massachusetts. The early generations of these mice segregated coat color, and were independently inbred to generate black mice (C57BL) and brown mice (C57BR).

Individual members of an inbred strain of mice are absolutely identical in their genetic makeup, and therefore they provide a resource from which identical animals can be used for studies where variations in genetic background must be avoided. The types of studies that have seen dramatic advances as a result of the development of inbred strains of mice include transplantation biology, cancer biology, and immunology, to name but a few.

C.   Congenic strains of mice

Before it became possible to experimentally introduce genes into mice, the idea of producing congenic strains of mice was developed. A congenic mouse is one which is genetically identical to an inbred strain of mice, with the exception of a gene and other closely-linked genes that have been purposely bred onto the inbred strain. The desired gene can be selected on the basis of phenotype, such as a coat color characteristic, a histocompatibility antigen, a gene that predisposes the animal towards autoimmune disease, or cancer susceptibility, as examples. In producing a congenic line of mice, however, the gene of interest is not the only gene that is selected for. All closely linked genes to the selected gene that are not removed by recombination during the breeding are also present in the new strain of mice. The amount of genetic material surrounding the selected gene that remains is therefore random and impossible to control.

A congenic line of mice is derived initially by mating two strains of animals, for example, C57BL/10 (a substrain of C57) and DBA/2 (also a substrain of DBA). If you want to breed a particular marker from the DBA/2 strain onto C57BL/10 mice, you would select the progeny from this mating (the F1 progeny) and backcross it to a C57BL/10 mouse. The offspring of this crossing would then be tested for the DBA/2 marker, and positive offspring would be bred to a C57BL/10 mouse again. By continuing this strategy of backcrossing, you would eventually select for a mouse whose genetic composition was derived from C57BL/10, but with the marker, and closely related genes, from the DBA/2 mouse. After 10 or more generations of backcrossing (the more, the better!), the backcrossed offspring with the DBA/2 marker are intercrossed and tested for homozygosity of the donor DBA/2 marker. This yields (in theory) a mouse homozygous for all genes from the parental C57BL/10 strain, except for the selected genes. These mice can then be inbred as the congenic strain of mice. In this particular example, the congenic strain of mice that was developed is called "B10.D2".

One investigator (Edward Golub) likened the production of a congenic strain of mice to making a very dry martini containing an olive, starting with a glass of vermouth containing an olive, and a bottle of gin. Mix the vermouth with an equal part of gin (the F1 generation). Remove half of the mix, and replace it with gin, always keeping the olive. Take this first "backcross" generation and repeat, always removing half of the mix, replacing it with gin, and keeping the olive. Eventually, you will have a glass with very little vermouth, but still containing the olive. Similarly, in producing congenic lines, each generation of backcrossing "dilutes out" the unwanted genes, without throwing out the gene of interest.

Table 5. Selected Nobel Laureates (The major histocompatibility complex and immune function)

Baruj Benacerraf Jean Dausset George D. Snell	discovery of the major histocompatibility complex; construction of congenic mice	1980[†]
Joseph E. Murray E. Donnall Thomas	development of organ transplantation	1990[†]
Peter C. Doherty Rolf M. Zinkernagel	elucidation of the role of the MHC in determining T cell specificity in cell mediated immunity	1996[†]

[†]Nobel Prize in Physiology or Medicine

Congenic strains of mice were instrumental in helping to understand the nature of genes that encode histocompatibility antigens and to define the Major Histocompatibility Complex (MHC). The MHC is called H-2 in mouse, and HLA in humans, and encodes a number of closely linked genes that are responsible for the rejection of tissues (kidneys, heart, skin, *etc.*) that are transplanted between two unrelated individuals. MHC differences trigger profound immunological responses, and are the reason that immunosuppressive drugs are required when transplanting tissues between any two persons except identical twins. These genes also help guide the development of receptors for foreign antigen on one of the major classes of lymphocytes, T lymphocytes. George Snell developed the idea of generating congenic mice for identifying the genes involved in tissue rejection, and for this work was awarded the Nobel Prize in 1980 (which he shared with Baruj Benacerraf and Jean Dausset) for the discovery and characterization of the MHC (Table 5).

Congenic strains of mice have also been used to determine the importance of a gene (and closely linked genes) to the onset of disease. They have also contributed significantly to studies that have mapped genes that contribute to complex diseases, such as systemic lupus erythematosis, an autoimmune disease that plagues hundreds of thousands of people, especially women. Generating and testing these mice takes patience: it can take three years or more to produce one individual mouse line.

Speed congenic strains of mice

Speed congenics utilize genomic scanning methods to help reduce the number of generations of backcrossing necessary to generate a congenic line. In this method, donor mice having the gene of interest are mated with a host strain of mice that can be distinguished on the basis of a large number of easily defined genetic polymorphisms. Frequently, differences called simple sequence length polymorphisms (SSLPs) are used for this purpose, since these can be identified rapidly by PCR. SSLPs are, as the name implies, differences in the number of base pairs of DNA found between two homologous regions between two different individuals. Because the genome of higher organisms has far more DNA than is required to code for the necessary genes, segments of DNA can be added, or subtracted, from noncoding regions without having any deleterious effect, giving rise to SSLPs.

In producing speed congenics, mice are screened after the first backcross generation for both the donor gene of interest AND identifiable polymorphisms between the two strains of mice. Those mice with the donor gene of interest, and the highest percentage of <u>host</u> markers, are then used for the next generation of backcrossing. This method reduces the number of generations of breeding by a factor of 2, thus reducing the time needed to produce the congenic line from 3 years to $1^1/_2$ years or less.

D.   Transgenic mice

Introduction

One of the most useful features of using mice in biomedical research is the ability to manipulate their genomes, either inserting genes or functionally deleting them. This has made it possible not only to investigate the properties of individual genes in the whole animal context (what do the genes do? how does it differ in different tissues?), but also to generate animal models for human diseases.

A transgenic organism is one in which foreign DNA has been integrated into their germ line (sperm or eggs, as opposed to somatic cells) by experimental introduction. Transgenics can be animals or plants. In the biomedical sciences, mice have been particularly amenable to transgenic technology. They have been used to study the regulation of gene function, the role of particular genes in cell development, and for the production of mouse models for human diseases, to name but a few. The first transgenic mouse was reported in 1980 by Gordon and Ruddle (43). The ability of the transgene to be transmitted in the germline was demonstrated the following year by a number of groups of investigators, including this one. From these first reports, barely 23 years ago, thousands of transgenic mouse lines have now been produced in many different laboratories.

Production of transgenic mice

To produce a transgenic mouse, DNA is injected into the pronucleus of a fertilized ovum (egg). In most transgenic models, DNA encoding the gene of interest, including regulatory (promoter and enhancer) regions surrounding the gene, is injected into the egg. The injected DNA is randomly integrated into the host DNA in some of the eggs; frequently multiple copies of the transgene are incorporated into a single integration site as a tandem array. The injected eggs are then re-implanted into "pseudopregnant" female mice, which was prepared by hormone treatment, and allowed to develop to full term. After birth, the DNA of the offspring is screened for the presence of the transgene, and positive mice are then bred (usually to an inbred strain of mice) to produce a transgenic line. Because not all mice that have incorporated a transgene will necessarily express it, mice are usually tested within 1 to 2 generations for expression of the transgene. Transgenic lines that express the gene will then be maintained for study.

In classic transgenic technology, transgenes are not integrated where the gene would normally be encoded. Therefore, the ability of the transgene to be expressed is often limited by a number of variables, including whether all of the gene's regulatory regions have been successfully cloned into the transgene. In addition, the site of integration can dramatically affect both the level of expression and the correct tissue specificity of expression of the transgene, since the site of integration may both inhibit or permit (or amplify) expression. For this reason, a number of independently derived transgenic lines are often produced and examined before selecting one or two for further studies.

BAC and YAC transgenics

Conventional transgenic mice are generated using purified DNA containing a gene's coding sequences and its regulatory elements. Such transgenes are generally limited to about 20,000 bp (20 kb) or less in size. Conventional transgenic approaches, therefore, cannot be used for genes that are encoded over larger regions of DNA, or have complex regulatory regions that control their expression or tissue specificity. Transgenic technology also cannot be used for the cloning and expression of linked genes that are encoded over larger stretches of DNA. As already mentioned, the correct tissue specific expression of conventional transgenes is subject to the site of integration. Some of these limitations of transgenic technology are overcome by incorporating significantly larger segments surrounding genes using artificial chromosomes, including BACs and YACs (described in Chapter 3).

Artificial chromosomes can be used to clone significantly larger stretches of DNA, as much as two million bp. The use of artificial chromosomes in constructing transgenic mice can be used for studies of linked genes, as well as for studies in which the correct spatial and temporal regulation of a gene(s) is required.

E.   Targeted transgenes: "knockout" and "knockin" mice

Targeted transgenic mice are special types of transgenics in which an endogenous gene is functionally or completely eliminated (knockout) or altered (knockin). The process for creating targeted transgenic mice is quite different than the method for creating transgenic mice. Instead of beginning with a fertilized ovum, targeted transgenes begin with embryonic stem cells (ES cells) and a modified genomic DNA construct called a targeting vector. The targeting vector is used to alter or replace the endogenous gene using the process of homologous recombination within the ES cell line. Homologous recombination is the process that results from the exchange of genetic material between two DNA molecules (usually paired chromosomes) at sites of DNA identity (homology). In the case of making targeted transgenics, one of the two "chromosomes" is replaced by the targeting vector carrying the alteration of interest.

ES cells are cells that have the capacity to give rise to all cells of the body. Human ES cells have recently received considerable attention in the press and in government due to their potential use for cloning human beings. The isolation and description of the first ES cells *in vitro* was reported by Martin Evans and Matt Kaufman in 1981 (44). Evans shared the Lasker Award for Biomedical Research in 2001 with Mario Capecchi (45,46) and Oliver Smithies (47,48) for their work on developing knockout technology. A number of Lasker Award winners have gone on to win Nobel Prizes of their own.

Knockout mice

Knockout mice are used to create models of human diseases in which genes have been silenced, such as Alzheimer's disease, cystic fibrosis, heart disease, and diseases caused by immunological defects. For generating knockout mice, the targeting vectors contain the gene of interest with variable amounts of flanking sequences (usually 1 to 10 kb). One or more exons of the gene are replaced by a selectable marker under the control of a constitutively active promoter. The selectable marker

Figure 11.   Production of a targeted transgenic by homologous recombination

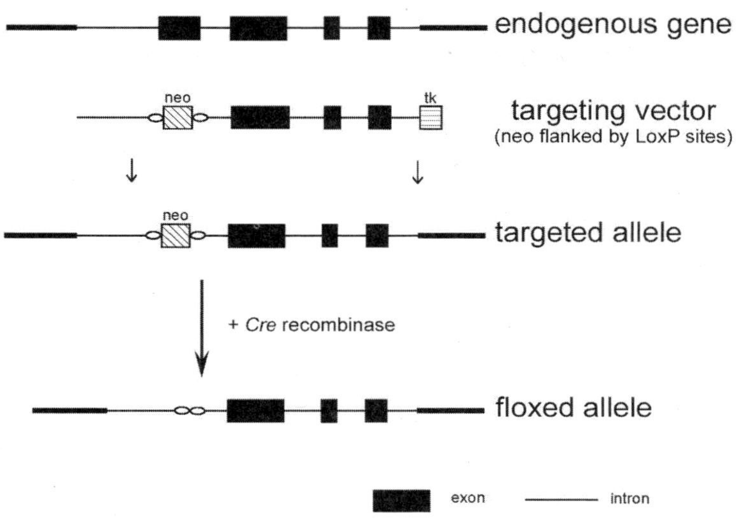

confers resistance to a drug that will otherwise kill the ES cells, such as the neomycin resistance gene (*neo*) which is commonly used for this purpose. Because homologous recombination is a rare event, the targeting construct often contains another selectable marker outside of the flanking regions of homology (Figure 11). This selectable marker is one which will kill ES cells that incorporate it into the DNA. A gene encoding a toxin, such as diphtheria toxin, can be used. Alternatively, a gene that confers sensitivity to a drug is often employed for negative selection. One example is the herpes simplex virus thymidine kinase (TK) gene, which confers sensitivity to the drug gancyclovir. By using a double selection system, cells that randomly incorporate the targeting vector as a transgene are eliminated, while cells that have incorporated it by homologous recombination are positively selected. Consequently, ES cells to be used for the next step in the process are rapidly identified.

The targeting construct is introduced into the ES cell line by electroporation, and the cells' enzymatic machinery does the magic. In ES cells that survive selection, the change in the endogenous gene is confirmed by Southern blot analysis. The modified ES cells are injected into blastocysts, an early stage in embryogenesis characterized by a sphere of cells enclosing an inner mass of cells in a fluid-filled cavity, which have been harvested from donor female mice. Several injected blastocysts are then implanted into the uterine horn of pseudopregnant recipient mice. If these survive to full term, they give rise to "chimeric" mice. Chimeric mice are mice that contain cells of more than one geno-type. The name chimera has its origins in Greek mythology and is taken from the Greek word meaning "she-goat". This mystical creature was the offspring of Echinda and Typhon and had the body of a goat, the head of a lion, and the tail of a serpent. Such chimeric creatures have often been represented in mythology. Other examples include centaurs, half horse and half man, the sphinx, with a human head on a lion's body, and the minotaur, which is half bull and half man. There is also a natural form of a chimera that exists in nature, and many cattle farmers will be familiar with it. Twin cattle share a placental membrane, and con-sequently there is an exchange of blood between the twins. When the twins are male and female, the female, called a "freemartin" is usually infertile: even though the animal is genetically female, it will have many male characteristics. But, I digress.

In constructing chimeric mice using ES cells, combinations of ES cells and donor blastocysts are used which derive from mice that differ in coat color. As a result, chimeric offspring are obvious since they contain coats that are not uniform in color, but are made up of the two different donor cells. The chimeric mice are then bred; if the ES cells have contributed to germ cells (sperm or egg), then offspring containing the modified gene will be obtained. These can be crossed to generate homozygous knockout mice.

Knockin mice

Knockin mice are generated in much the same way. The only real difference is that instead of being designed to eliminate an endogenous gene, the targeting construct is made so that the endogenous gene will be altered. For example, coding sequences can be mutated in order to generate a mouse model of a human mutation, or regulatory sequences can be changed in order to alter the expression of a gene. Alternatively, the endogenous mouse gene can be replaced by its human counterpart.

Floxed genes in knockout technology

Although knockouts were originally generated using genes in which an exon(s) had been replaced by the *neo* gene, it became clear that this gene, and its accompanying promoter, could introduce artifacts of its own. Consequently, a method to eliminate the *neo* marker was devel-oped. This takes advantage of a P1 bacteriophage recombinase, *Cre*, and its binding sites, *loxP*. *LoxP* sites are 34 bp sequences with an 8 bp core sequence (that determines directionality of the recombina-tion event), and flanked by 13 bp palindromic sequences. When a DNA sequence, such as that containing the *neo* gene, is flanked by *LoxP* sites (flanked *LoxP* sites are "floxed"), addition of the *Cre* recombinase results in its deletion. To remove the intervening sequences flanked by *loxP* sites in ES cells, a vector containing the *Cre* recombinase can be introduced into the ES cells by electroporation. Figure 11 shows the removal of the selectable neo gene using this technology.

Conditional mutants using floxed genes

The use of the Cre-lox system has now evolved well beyond its initial use in removing the selectable marker from targeting vectors in ES cells. Today, this system is used to delete genes in an inducible or tissue specific fashion to conditionally delete genes. This technology is especially useful in the studies of genes that affect development, since knockouts of these genes often lead to embryonic lethality. To generate conditional mutants, two different approaches are used.

In the first approach, two different transgenic mouse lines are independently generated, one carrying the *Cre* recombinase under the control of a tissue specific promoter, and a second carrying the floxed gene. The two strains of mice are mated. The floxed gene is deleted in the progeny mice, but only in the tissues in which the *Cre* recombinase is expressed. Currently, there are a number of *Cre* transgenic mouse lines that express the recombinase under the control of different promoters that have very selective tissue specificity.

A second approach utilizes mice in which the *Cre* recombinase is under the expression of an inducible promoter. In these systems, floxed genes are deleted only when the inducible promoter is activated, therefore activating the expression of the recombinase. This is especially useful if the investigator wishes to delete a gene only after it has been expressed, as a means to determine the role that particular gene product plays after the development of a tissue. Inducible promoters that have been used for these purposes include response elements that are activated by antibiotics, such as tetracycline, or hormone analogues, such as tamoxifen (the estrogen antagonist that is used for the treatment and prevention of breast cancer).

The FLP-FRT system

The FLP-FRT system is very similar to the Cre-lox system and is becoming increasingly popular in the generation of knockout mice, either alone or in combination with the Cre-lox system. FLP is a flippase recombinase isolated for the yeast *Saccharomyces cerevisiae*, and FRT is the flippase recombination target sequence. When genes are flanked by FRT sites, the addition of the FLP results in their deletion (as long as the orientation of the sequences is appropriate, like the *loxP* sites).

RAG-deficient blastocyst complementation

RAG-1 and RAG-2 (recombination activating genes 1 and 2) are lymphoid specific enzymes that are required for the production of antigen-specific receptors on T and B lymphocytes. In the absence of either of these genes, lymphocytes do not develop. Mutations in RAG-1 or RAG-2 are one of several defects that lead to the syndrome called severe combined immunodeficiency (SCID). Children who are born with this disease usually die of infections within 2 to 3 years after birth. Mutant mice that lack one or the other of these genes have been created by knockout technology. In addition to allowing for the study of the role these enzymes play in production of lymphocytes, these mice can be used for the creation of chimeric mice for the study of gene function in lymphocyte development (49).

RAG-2-deficient blastocyst complementation uses blastocysts from RAG-2 deficient mice. These are injected with modified ES cells, in which the gene of interest has been inactivated or mutated, and implanted into mice for development. Any lymphocytes that develop in the offspring will have developed from the ES cells, since the RAG-2-deficient cells cannot give rise to these lineages. Any mutations that have been introduced in the ES cells can therefore be screened for their affect on T and B lymphocyte development and function.

F.   Other uses of mice in biomedical research

N-ethyl-N-nitrosourea (ENU) mutagenesis

ENU is a powerful chemical mutagen that creates random single point mutations in the genome. It is now used for genome-wide mutagenesis studies in mice, a concept first proven to be useful for a variety of genetic analysis in lower organisms, including fruit flies and nematodes. ENU is such a powerful mutagen that it can be used to identify genes that are involved in complex genetic traits in the mouse. ENU is used to mutagenize spermatogonia in male mice. Once mature sperm develop from the spermatogonia, the males are mated with untreated female mice, and offspring are evaluated for the function in which the investigator is interested. Both dominant mutations and recessive mutations can be detected by this methodology, although recessive mutations require additional breeding in order to obtain animals that are homozygous for the recessive allele. Although it is time consuming and expensive, the value of this approach is that it can be used to target, in theory, every gene in the body. In addition, the generation of point mutations often results in phenotypes that are different from those that are revealed in gene deletion in knockout mice, since protein products are usually made carrying the mutations. This can make it more difficult for other gene products to compensate for the affected gene.

Bone marrow chimeras

Bone marrow chimeras, also known as radiation chimeras or tetra-parental mice, are mice that have had all of their hematopoietic cells replaced using bone marrow stem cells from other mice. This is a common tool that is used in immunologic studies. Recipient mice are lethally irradiated (hence the name "radiation" chimera), which destroys all of the progenitor cells in the bone marrow, including pleuripotent stem cells. They are then reconstituted with bone marrow cells from donor animals, which survive indefinitely, as well as give rise to committed progenitor cells that differentiate to form all of the blood elements, including erythrocytes (red blood cells), lymphocytes, monocytes, neutrophils, platelets, *etc*. These mice will then be permanently reconstituted with the blood cells from another animal. Consequently, they are referred to as "tetra-parental" (yes, four parents.) chimeras.

Adoptive transfer

Adoptive transfer is a method in which immune cells (lymphocytes) from one mouse are used to provide immunity to an antigen or pathogen to another mouse. To perform an adoptive transfer experiment, recipient mice are sublethally irradiated (350R to 450R versus the lethal dose of irradiation required to totally eliminate stem cells from the bone marrow, which ranges from 850R to 1100R). Sublethal irradiation temporarily depletes lymphocytes from secondary lymphoid organs (spleen and lymph nodes), which provides room for the cells to be transferred. In contrast to the production of bone marrow chimeras, in an adoptive transfer experiment mature cells, usually lymphocytes and often from an immune donor, are transferred into recipient mice. Because these cells have limited lifespan and do not (normally) repopulate themselves, the chimeric state that is achieved in adoptive transfer experiments is short-lived.

References

1. Lowry, O. H., N. J. Rosebrough, A. L. Farr, and R. J. Randall. 1951. Protein measurement with the folin phenol reagent. *J. Biol. Chem.* 193: 265–275.

2. Bradford, M. M. 1976. A rapid and sensitive method for the quantitation of microgram quantities of protein utilizing the principle of protein-dye binding. *Anal. Biochem.* 72: 248–254.

3. Studier, F. W. 2000. Slab-gel electrophoresis. *Trends Biochem. Sci.* 25: 588–590.

4. Maizel, J. V. 2000. SDS polyacrylamide gel electrophoresis. *Trends Biochem. Sci.* 25: 590–592.

5. Laemmli U. K. 1970. cleavage of structural proteins during the assembly of the head of bacteriophage T4. *Nature* 227: 680–685.

6. Summers, D. F., J. V. Maizel Jr., and J. E. Darnell Jr. 1965. Evidence for virus-specific noncapsid proteins in poliovirus-infected HeLa cells. *Proc. Natl. Acad. Sci. USA* 54: 505–513.

7. Towbin, H., T. Staehelin, and J. Gordon. 1979. Electrophoretic transfer of proteins from polyacrylamide gels to nitrocellulose sheets: procedure and some applications. *Proc. Natl. Acad. Sci. USA* 76: 4350–4354.

8. Fields, S. and O.-K. Song. 1989. A novel genetic system to detect protein-protein interactions. *Nature* 340: 245–246.

9. Watson, J. D. and F. H. C. Crick. 1953. Molecular structure of nucleic acids. A structure of deoxyribose nucleic acid. *Nature* 171: 737–738.

10. Avery, O. T., C. M. MacLeod, and M. McCarty. 1944. Studies on the chemical nature of the substance inducing transformation of pneumococcal types. Induction of transformation by a desoxyribonucleid acid fraction isolated from Pneumococcus Type III. *J. Exp. Med.* 79: 137–158.

11. Danna, K. and D. Nathans. 1971. Specific cleavage of simian virus 40 DNA by restriction endonuclease of Hemophilus influenzae. *Proc. Natl. Acad. Sci. USA* 68: 2913–2917.

12. Kelly, T. J. Jr. and H. O. Smith. 1970. A restriction enzyme from Hemophilus influenzae. II. *J. Mol. Biol.* 51: 393–409.

13. Botstein, D., R. L. White, M. Skolnick, and R. W. Davis. 1980. Construction of a genetic linkage map in man using restriction fragment length polymorphisms. *Am. J. Hum. Genet.* 32: 314–331.

14. Southern, E. M. 1975. Detection of specific sequences among DNA fragments separated by gel electrophoresis. *J. Mol. Biol.* 98: 503–518.

15. Maxam, A. M. and W. Gilbert. 1977. A new method for sequencing DNA. *Proc. Natl. Acad. Sci. USA* 74: 560–564.

16. Sanger, F., S. Nicklen, and A. R. Coulson. 1977. DNA sequencing with chain-terminating inhibitors. *Proc. Natl. Acad. Sci. USA* 74: 5463–5467.

17. Alwine, J. C., D. J. Kemp, B. A. Parker, J. Reiser, J. Renart, G. R. Stark, and G. M. Wahl. 1979. Detection of specific RNAs or specific fragments of DNA by fractionation in gels and transfer to diazobenzyloxymethyl paper. *Methods Enzymol.* 68: 220–242.

18. Baltimore, D. 1970. RNA-dependent DNA polymerase in virions of RNA tumour viruses. *Nature* 226: 1209–1211.

19. Goff, S. P. and P. Berg. 1976. Construction of hybrid viruses containing SV40 and lambda phage DNA segments and their propagation in cultured monkey cells. *Cell* 9: 695–705.

20. Huynh, T. V., R. A. Young, and R. W. Davis. 1985. Constructing and screening cDNA libraries in λgt10 and λgt11. *DNA Cloning: A Practical Approach* 1: 49–78.

21. Frischauf, A. M., H. Lehrach, A. Poustka, and N. Murray. 1983. Lambda replacement vectors carrying polylinker sequences. *J. Mol. Biol.* 170: 827–842.

22. Hutchison, C. A. 3rd, S. Phillips M. H. Edgell, S. Gillam, P. Jahnke, and M. Smith. 1978. Mutagenesis at a specific position in a DNA sequence. *J. Biol. Chem.* 253; 6551–6560.

23. Saiki, R. K., S. Scharf, F. Faloona, K. B. Mullis, G. T. Horn, H. A. Erlich, and N. Arnheim. 1985. Enzymatic amplification of beta-globin genomic sequences and restriction site analysis for diagnosis of sickle cell anemia. *Science* 230: 1350–1354.

24. Mullis, K. B. 1990. The unusual origin of the polymerase chain reaction. *Sci. Am.* 262: 56–65.

25. Higuchi, R., G. Dollinger, P. S. Walsh, and R. Griffith. 1992. Simultaneous amplification and detection of specific DNA sequences. *Biotechnology* 10: 413–417.

26. Adams, M. D., J. M. Kelley, J. D. Gocayne, M. Dubnick, M. H. Polymeropoulos, H. Xiao, C. R. Merril, A. Wu, B. Olde, R. F. Moreno, and et al. 1991. Complementary DNA sequencing: expressed sequence tags and human genome project. *Science* 252: 1651–1656.

27. Garner, M. M. and A. Revzin. 1981. A gel electrophoresis method for quantifying the binding of proteins to specific DNA regions: application to components of the E. coli lactose operon regulating system. *Nucl. Acids Res.* 9: 3047–3060.

28. Foster, E. A., M. A. Jobling, P. G. Tayler, P. Donnelly, P. de Knijff, R. Mieremet, T. Zerjal, and C. Tyler-Smith. 1998. Jefferson fathered slave's last child. *Nature* 396: 27–28.

29. Köhler, G. and C. Milstein. 1975. Continuous cultures of fused cells secreting antibody of predetermined specificity. *Nature* 256: 495–497.

30. Kessler, S. W. 1975. Rapid isolation of antigens from cells with a staphylococcal protein A-antibody adsorbent: parameters of the interaction of antibody-antigen complexes with protein A. *J. Immunol.* 115: 1617–1624.

31. Coons, A. H., H. J. Creech, and R. N. Jones. 1941. Immunological properties of an antibody containing a fluorescent group. *Proc. Soc. Expt. Biol. Med.* 47: 200–202.

32. Yalow, R. S. and S. A. Breson. 1960. Immunoassay of endogenous plasma insulin in man. *J. Clin. Invest.* 39: 1157–1175.

33. Engvall, E. and P. Perlman. 1971. Enzyme-linked immunosorbent assay (ELISA). Quantitative assay of immunoglobulin G. *Immunochemistry* 8: 871–874.

34. Jerne, N. K. and A. A. Nordin. 1963. Plaque formation in agar by single antibody-producing cells. *Science* 140: 405.

35. Coons, A. H., H. J. Creech, N. Jones, and E. Berliner. 1942. The demonstration of pneumococcal antigen in tissues by the use of fluorescent antibody. *J. Immunol.* 45: 159–170.

36. White, J. G., W. B. Amos, and M. Fordham. 1987. An evaluation of confocal versus conventional imaging of biological structures by fluorescence light microsocopy. *J. Cell Biol.* 105: 41–48.

37. Agard, D. A. and J. W. Sedat. 1983. Three-dimensional architecture of a polytene nucleus. *Nature* 302: 676–681.

38. Knoll, M. and E. Ruska. 1932. Das Elektronemikroskop. *Z. Physik* 78: 318–339.

39. Klug, A. and J. E. Berger. 1964. An optical method for the analysis of periodicities in electron micrographs, and some observations on the mechanism of negative staining. *J. Mol. Biol.* 10: 565–569.

40. Damadian, R. 1971. Tumor detection by nuclear magnetic resonance. *Science* 171: 1151–1153.

41. Lauterbur, P. 1973. Image formation by induced local interactions: examples employing nuclear magnetic resonance. *Nature* 242: 190–191.

42. Mansfield, P. and P. K. Grannell. 1973. NMR 'diffraction' in solids? *J. Phys. C: Solid State Phys.* 6: L422–L426.

43. Gordon, J. W., G. A. Scangos, D. J. Plotkin, J. A. Barbosa, and F. H. Ruddle. 1980. Genetic transformation of mouse embryos by microinjection of purified DNA. *Proc. Natl. Acad. Sci. USA* 77: 7380–7384.

44. Evans, M. J. and M. H. Kaufman. 1981. Establishment in culture of pluripotential cells from mouse embryos. *Nature* 292: 154–156.

45. Mansour, S. L., K. R. Thomas, and M. R. Capecchi. 1988. Disruption of the proto-oncogene int-2 in mouse embryo-derived stem cells: a general strategy for targeting mutations to non-selectable genes. *Nature* 336: 348–352.

46. Thomas, K. R. And M. R. Capecchi. 1990. Targeted disruption of the murine int-1 proto-oncogene resulting in severe abnormalities in midbrain and cerebellar development. *Nature* 346: 847–850.

47. Koller, B. H. and O. Smithies. 1989. Inactivating the beta 2-microglobulin locus in mouse embryonic stem cells by homologous recombination. *Proc. Natl. Acad. Sci. USA* 86: 8932–8935.

48. Koller, B. H., L. J. Hagemann, T. Doetschman, J. R. Hagaman, S. Huang, P. J. Williams, N. L. First, N. Maeda, and O. Smithies. 1989. Germ-line transmission of a planned alteration made in a hypoxanthine phosphoribosyltransferase gene by homologous recombination in embryonic stem cells. *Proc. Natl. Acad. Sci. USA* 86: 8927–8931.

49. Chen, J., R. Lansford, V. Stewart, F. Young, and F. W. Alt. 1993. RAG-2-deficient blastocyst complementation: an assay of gene function in lymphocyte development. *Proc. Natl. Acad. Sci. USA* 90: 4528–4532.

Some excellent methodology manuals

Russell, D.W. and J. Sambrook. 2001. **Molecular Cloning: A Laboratory Manual.** J. Argentine, editor. Cold Spring Harbor Laboratory Press, New York (3 volumes).

Harlow, E. and D. Lane. 1999. **Using Antibodies: A Laboratory Manual.** Cold Spring Harbor Laboratory Press, New York.

The following manuals are all published by John Wiley & Sons and remain current as they are updated several times each year.

Ausubel, F.M., R. Brent, R.E. Kingston, D.D. Moore, J.G. Seidman, J.A. Smith, and K. Struhl, editors. **Current Protocols in Molecular Biology** (4 volumes; a.k.a. *the Red Book*).

Coligan, J.E., A.M. Kruisbeek D.H. Margulies, E.M. Shevach, and W. Strober, editors. **Current Protocols in Immunology** (4 volumes; a.k.a. *the Gold Book*).

Bonifacino, J.S., M. Dasso, J.B. Harford, J. Lippincott-Schwartz, and K.M. Yamada, editors. **Current Protocols in Cell Biology** (2 volumes; a.k.a. *the Green Book*).

Coligan J.E., B.M. Dunn, H.L. Ploegh, D.W. Speicher, and P.T. Wingfield, editors. **Current Protocols in Protein Science** (3 volumes; a.k.a. *the Blue Book*).

Index